5-Ingredient Clean-Eating Cookbook

Over 50 Easy Few-Ingredients Recipes for Fast and Healthy Cooking. Part 3.

Cooking time – from 5 minutes

By Karla Bro

Copyright © 2021 by Karla Bro

All rights reserved.

No part of this book may be reproduced or transmitted in any form or by any means, electronic or mechanical, including photocopying, recording, or any information storage and retrieval system, without permission in writing from the publisher.

Disclaimer

All material in " 5-Ingredient Clean-Eating Cookbook. Over 50 Easy Few-Ingredients Recipes for Fast and Healthy Cooking. Part 3. Cooking time – from 5 minutes" is provided for your information only and may not be construed as medical advice or instruction. No action or inaction should be taken based solely on the contents of this information. Consult appropriate professionals for your health and well-being.

Remember that cooking is subjective. You may not achieve the desired results due to different brands of ingredients or different cooking abilities. Avoid your allergens.

I am not a chef. I'm just a person who likes cooking and writing about home-cooked food. Most of my recipes are created based on personal taste.

Table of Contents

LITTLE CHANGES ARE THE WAY TO A HEALTHIER LIFE 6

WHAT IS CLEAN-EATING DIET 7

HOW TO TRANSITIONS TO A CLEAN DIET 8

CLEAN EATING RULES 10

CLEAN NUTRITION HAS MANY ADVANTAGES 13

BREAKFAST 14

    Breakfast Sweet Potatoes 15

    Curry Scrambled Eggs 16

    Nectarine and Beet Salad 17

    Breakfast Banana Splits 19

    Pomegranates and Grapefruit Breakfast with Honey-Yogurt Sauce 20

    Almond Cherry Smoothie by Natalie Coughlin 22

    Strawberry Banana Smoothie 23

    Mexican Egg Scramble 25

    1-Minute Eggs 26

    Poached Eggs 27

    Welsh Eggs 28

    Tea Oatmeal 30

    Tropical Oatmeal 31

    Egg Whites with Asparagus 32

    Oatmeal with Cardamom and Raisins 33

    Banana Split 35

    Carrot, Apple, and Orange Salad 36

    Amaranth Porridge 37

    Zucchini Omelette 38

    Eggs in Tomatoes 40

Flax Seed Smoothie 41

Roll-Up Omelet with Spinach 42

Tomato and Bell Pepper Smoothies 43

Tomato and Avocado Frittata 44

LUNCH AND DINNER 45

Black Bean Soup 46

Lentil Lasagne 47

Zucchini Fritters 48

Roasted Corn and Tilapia 50

Buttermilk Chicken 53

Shredded Kale and Brussels Sprouts Salad 54

Nicoise Salad with Asparagus 55

Warm Garlic Greens 57

Chicken Pesto Roll-Ups 58

Roasted Beet Wedges 60

Grilled Eggplant 62

Braised Beef and Zucchini 63

Coconut Chicken Strips 64

Pecan Butter with Brussels Sprouts 65

Boiled Chicken Breast with Rosemary 68

Salmon Spinach Pasta 69

Chicken & Celery Root Tikka Masala 70

Stuffed Potato and Hummus Dressing 73

Chicken Fillet with Salsa Sauce 74

Squash Boats with Pesto Spaghetti 75

5-Ingredient Quinoa Mac and Cheese 77

Stuffed Bell Pepper with Tomato and Chicken 78

DESSERTS	80
Flourless Chocolate Cookies	81
Banana Ice Cream	82
Berries and Cream Popsicles	83
Vegan Fudgsicles	84
Peanuts Coconuts Bites	86
Chocolate Bites	87
Cinnamon Pecan Cookies	88
Banana Bread Bites	90
Clean Eating Banoffee Parfaits	91
Mango and Cinnamon	93
Mini Fruit Pizzas	94
Apple "Donuts"	96
Birthday Cake Popcorn	97
Watermelon-Strawberry Popsicles	98
Banana Tarts	100
Ginger-Berry Dessert	101
Lemon Cheesecake	102
Pumpkin Cheesecake Mousse	104
Tropical Fruits Salad	105
Vegan Chocolate Turron	106
Coconut Snowballs	107

LITTLE CHANGES ARE THE WAY TO A HEALTHIER LIFE

Your food can become your friend. It can affect your health and the risk of certain diseases. If you want to be healthier, change your daily habits. Just try to do this. I don't mean huge changes. It will be helpful to change your life step by step. Over time, these small changes will make your life healthier.

Try to:

- Keep more vegetables and fruits
- Choose low-fat and whole-grain products
- Add healthy food, rather than removing unhealthy meals
- Take healthy food to work; in this way, you can control what you eat
- Don't delay and skip meals; don't ignore your feelings of hunger
- Eat your meal with others
- Drink water

And try to use this healthy recipe book and cook according to its instructions. Cooking will not take long in this case because there are no more than five ingredients in our recipes.

WHAT IS CLEAN-EATING DIET

Someone said that clean eating means abstaining from all processed food or eating only raw food. But this isn't true. Clean eating means rejecting products with a high degree of processing (fried products, chips, sweets). It is the consumption of whole, minimally processed (and even better generally unprocessed) food (brown rice, fruits, and vegetables). Instead of focusing on using a certain number of food groups (for example, fewer carbohydrates and more protein), the idea of pure nutrition revolves around being attentive to food processing. The focus of a clean diet is the consumption of whole foods in their natural (if possible) or least-processed state, in which a significant amount of nutrients are retained during processing.

There are many problems associated with highly processed foods: excessive weight gain, the risk of cardiovascular diseases. Products with a high degree of processing don't have the nutrients necessary to maintain your overall health. Most of what you get from these foods are "empty" calories without the right amount of protein and trace elements. The result of this diet is a lack of nutrients, which predisposes you to various diseases.

HOW TO TRANSITIONS TO A CLEAN DIET

1. ***The decision should be well thought out and not just emotional.*** So, determine the reason and tell yourself, "That's why I turned to clean food, and I am not going to turn off my intended path!"
2. ***Allocate time.*** Sit down and think about how much time you can devote to a new lifestyle. You may have to spend an extra hour a day preparing a healthy lunch.
3. ***Goals should be measurable and straightforward.*** If you love cookies, telling yourself, "I will eat fewer cookies" is abstract. Saying, "I will eat one cookie a day," is more specific, but it is better to say, "Instead of cookies, I will eat fruit."
4. ***Get rid of harmful products.*** List all your favorite "harmful" products. You need to throw away artificial, ultra-processed foods from your refrigerator and pantry.
5. ***Replenish your stocks with "clean" products.*** Gradually replace harmful products with clean products. Start with fruits and vegetables. Then include whole grain food in your diet.
6. ***Start your day with a fresh breakfast.*** Fruit and green smoothies are a good option. Eat this way for 1-2 weeks, and you'll develop the desire to eat clean lunches and dinners.
7. ***Do not eat when you are full.*** Do you not know proper portions? Stop eating when your stomach is full.
8. ***Study labels and choose products with natural ingredients.***

9. ***Get to know your local farmers.*** They will be able to supply you with independently grown, organic products.
10. ***Start cooking.***
11. ***Adhere to the clean food plan.*** Count the calories

If you want to lose weight, reduce your number of calories and increase your physical activity. If you wish to lose 1 to 1 ½ pound per week, reduce your daily calorie intake by 500-750 calories:

- ***A diet with 1200 to 1500 calories per day is safe for women;***
- ***A diet with 1500 to 1800 calories per day is safe for men and women who exercise regularly.***

Don't use low-calorie diets of ***fewer than 800 calories per day.*** You can only eat in this way if your doctor is monitoring you.

CLEAN EATING RULES

Shopping

First, go to the grocery store and pay attention to the signs in the produce section about how far your fruits, veggies, meat, and fish had to travel to reach you. Read nutrition labels, and don't choose products with unknown ingredients. Instead, try to pick foods without boxes, cans, bags, and packaging. All the food must be fresh.

Cooking

Cook at home, and you will know all about salt and sugar in your meal. Don't use high-fat cooking methods, such as deep-frying or stewing with animal or vegetable fat. You can steam, bake, or grill. Use olive oil, replace salt with garlic, spices, herbs, and lemon.

Whole Grains and Natural Sugars

Try to complete your meal with whole grains. Choose legumes and beans. They will be beneficial for your heart. Natural sugar must be in your meal plan. Use honey, maple sugar, or dehydrated sugar cane juice. There is no fat, cholesterol in the organic sweeteners.

You can eat the following:

- Single-ingredient grains (farro, oats, barley, brown rice, quinoa, millet, and amaranth)

- Whole-wheat pasta

- Popcorn

- Sprouted whole-grain bread
- Whole-wheat pizza dough

Protein

Don't forget about protein, a vital muscle-builder. It's essential in the first part of the day. Make sure to eat proteins at breakfast and lunch. Clean proteins are these:

- Chicken breasts and legs, ground beef
- Seafood, such as wild salmon and Pacific cod
- Eggs
- Unflavored nuts, such as almonds, hazelnuts, cashews, and walnuts
- Plain nut butter without sugar
- Dried beans

Fruits and Vegetables

These products are always a clear choice. Don't worry about sugar content. It's hard to overdo it. Tasty fruits and useful vegetables contain a lot of fiber, vitamins, and minerals.

It's better to limit your consumption of fruit juice because even 100% fruit juice doesn't contain the whole fruits' beneficial fiber.

It's better to choose these:

- Fresh fruit
- Canned fruit without sugar

- Frozen fruit without sugar
- Dried fruit without sugar

Vegetables are the building blocks of clean-eating meals. They contain a lot of vitamins, minerals, and fiber. Canned and frozen vegetables are healthy too, but choose ones without sauces and read the labels.

Choose these vegetables:

- Any fresh vegetables
- Frozen and canned vegetables without sauce or salt.

Dairy

It's better to choose non-dairy alternatives than dairy products. Choices are coconut, soy, and almond milk. If you like dairy products, use regular or Greek yogurt, choose unsweetened varieties and low-fat products. Whole-milk dairy is the best choice.

Choose the following:

- Plain yogurt
- Milk
- Cheese
- Unsweetened non-dairy milk

CLEAN NUTRITION HAS MANY ADVANTAGES

HELP GET RID OF EXTRA WEIGHT, as documented by several studies. Lack of calories with a balanced diet allows your body to switch from fat storage mode to burning mode. At the same time, there is no deficiency of nutrients and no constant hunger because, in such food, there is a high content of micronutrients and protein. Protein is an essential nutrient for weight loss. It not only accelerates your metabolism but also reduces hunger. Additionally, more soluble fiber is in whole foods. Soluble fiber has many health benefits, one of which is increased weight loss.

REDUCES THE RISK OF CANCER DEVELOPMENT. Studies have shown a positive correlation between nutrition and the prevention of various types of cancer, including breast cancer and colon cancer.

REDUCES THE RISK OF HIGH BLOOD PRESSURE AND HEART DISEASES. These diseases are usually associated with high levels of bad cholesterol, but this problem can be eliminated by merely switching to a clean diet.

IMPROVES IMMUNITY. By eating five or more servings of fruits and vegetables per day, the body's immune response can be improved up to 82 percent.

IMPROVES SKIN CONDITION. Do not spend hundreds of dollars on cosmetics. Whole foods contain large amounts of antioxidants, healthy fats, and other nutrients that play a huge role in skin health.

BREAKFAST

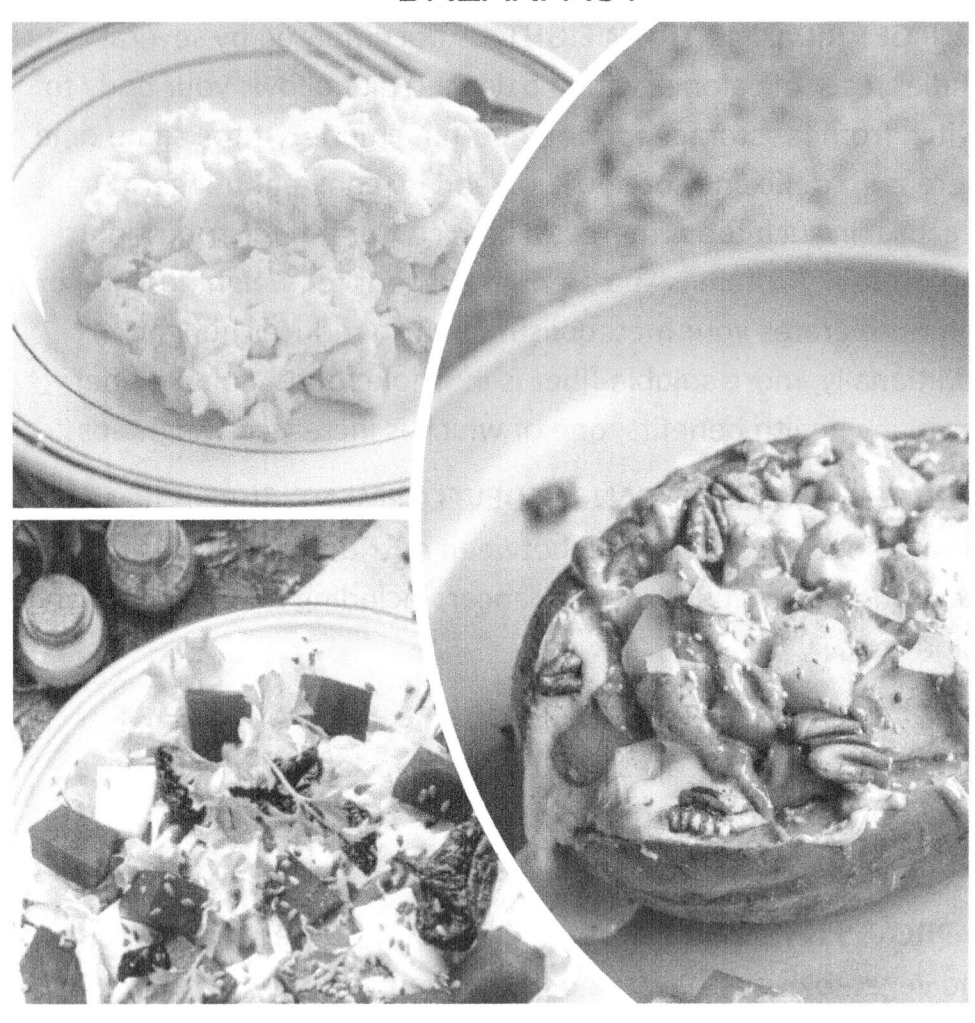

Breakfast Sweet Potatoes

Cooking time 55 min | Servings 4

Ingredients

4 medium sweet potatoes, 32 ounces

1/2 cup coconut Greek yogurt, fat-free

1 medium apple, chopped

2 tbsp maple syrup

1/4 cup toasted unsweetened coconut flakes

Use the nuts optional

Directions

1. Preheat oven to 400°F.
2. Peel and cut potatoes, place on a foil-lined baking sheet.
3. Bake the potatoes for 45-60 minutes until tender.
4. At the same time, chop the apple.
5. After baking, take the potatoes and cut an "X" in each piece. Take the fork and fluff pulp.
6. Mix apple, yogurt, maple syrup, and coconut flakes in a bowl. Top the potatoes with this mixture.

Nutrition facts per serving, 1 stuffed potato: 321 calories, 3g fat, 70g carbohydrate, 7g protein.

Curry Scrambled Eggs

Cooking time 15 min | Servings 4

Ingredients

8 large eggs

1/4 cup fat-free milk

1/2 tsp curry powder

1/4 tsp salt

1/8 tsp pepper

1/8 tsp ground cardamom, to taste

Directions

1. Take a large bowl. Add eggs, milk, salt, pepper, and curry powder, cardamom to it. Blend all ingredients.
2. Take a large non-stick skillet, grease it lightly—Preheat the skillet over medium heat. Pour egg mixture into the skillet. Cook the mixture and stir until thickened.
3. Slice the tomatoes and serve the eggs.

Nutrition facts per serving: 160 calories, 10g fat, 4g carbohydrate, 14g protein.

Nectarine and Beet Salad

Cooking time 10 min| Servings 8

Ingredients

10 oz mix salad greens

2 medium nectarines

1/4 cup balsamic vinegar

14.5 oz canned beets

1/2 cup crumbled feta cheese

Directions

1. Slice the nectarines, drained beets.
2. Take a big dish for serving. Toss greens, nectarines on it. Sprinkle the ingredients with vinaigrette.
3. Top the dish with beets and cheese.

Nutrition facts per serving: 69 calories, 3.14g fat, 6g carbohydrate, 3.25g protein.

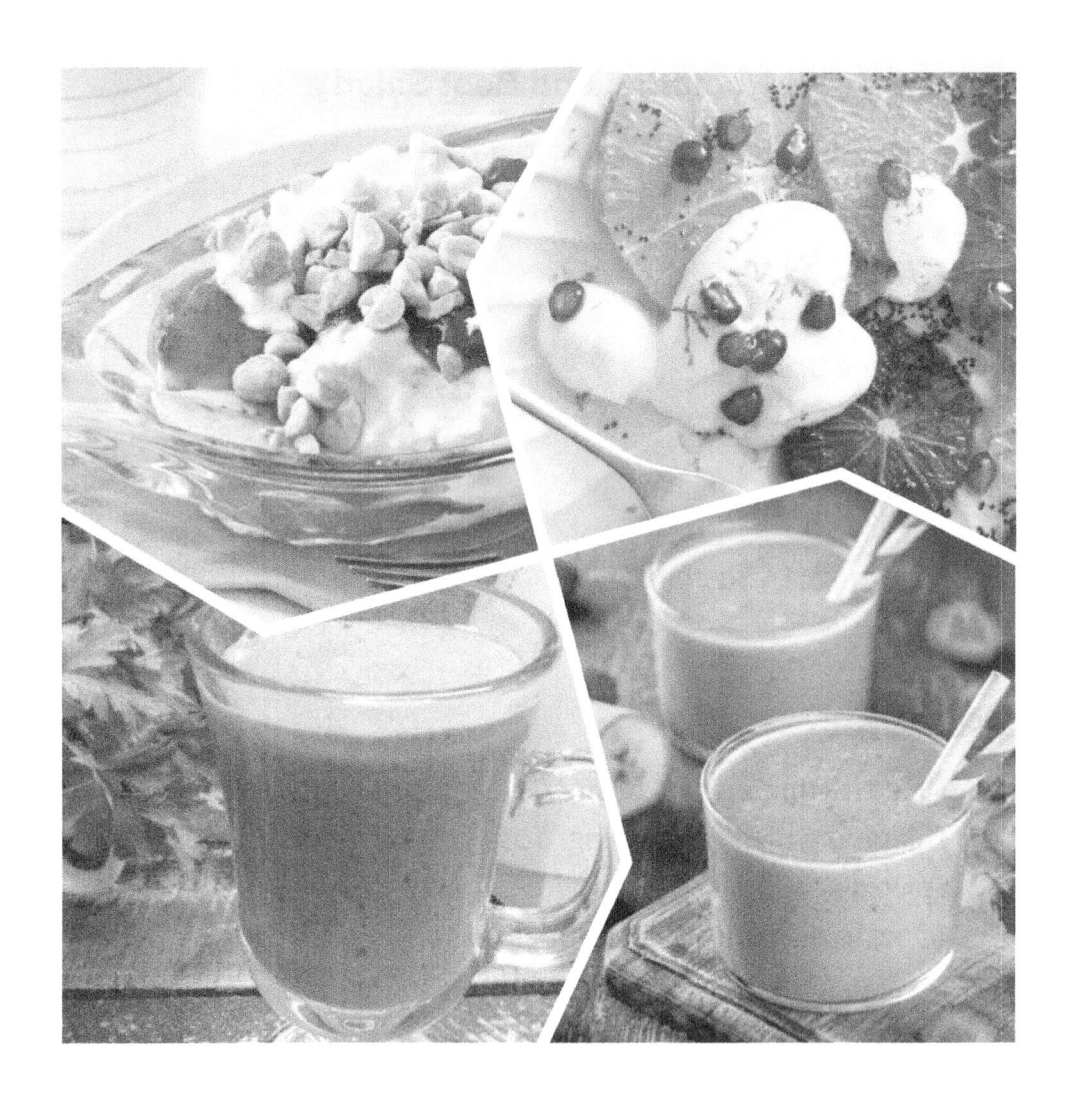

Breakfast Banana Splits

Cooking time 10 min | Servings 4

Ingredients

4 medium bananas

2 cups cottage cheese

6 tbsp all-fruit strawberry jam

1/4 cup roasted peanuts, chopped

1/8 tsp sea salt

Directions

1. Peel and cut each banana in half lengthwise.
2. Place eight banana halves in a bowl. Take a spoon or ice-cream scooper. Put the cottage cheese over the banana center, top with jam, 1.5 tbsp on each piece, add 1 tbsp peanuts, a pinch of salt.

Nutrition Facts per one banana split: 255 Calories, 44g carbohydrates, 6g fat, 17g protein.

Pomegranates and Grapefruit Breakfast with Honey-Yogurt Sauce

Cooking time 15 min | Servings 4

Ingredients

1 large pomegranate

1 large grapefruit

1 large orange

1/4 cup plain Greek yogurt, non-fat

1 tbsp raw honey

Optional 2 tbsp natural unsalted pine nuts, slivered almonds, or macadamia nuts

Directions

1. Pour water into a large bowl. Set the bowl aside.
2. Seed the pomegranate, add the seeds to the bowl.
3. Take the grapefruits, peel fruits. Cut the pomegranate into segments, discard the peel and pith.
4. Add the grapefruits to the water with pomegranate arils. Combine the ingredients gently.
5. Take a small bowl, pour honey and yogurt in it. Stir the ingredients well until creamy.
6. Place a medium skillet on medium heat. Toast in it nuts for 2-3 minutes. Shake skillet, toast until golden nuts and fragrant.

7. Remove the skillet from the heat and cool for 1 minute.
8. Dry the fruits, place them on the servings plates. Pour yogurt sauce on the top of the fruits, sprinkle with the nuts.

Nutritional facts per serving: 125 calories, 26g carbohydrates, 2g fat, 4g protein.

Almond Cherry Smoothie by Natalie Coughlin

Cooking time 5 min| Servings 2

Ingredients

1 cup almond milk, unsweetened

1 tbsp chia seeds

1/2 frozen banana

1 cup frozen dark cherries

1 tbsp almond butter

Directions

Place all ingredients in a food processor. Blend until smooth. Enjoy!

Nutritional facts per serving: 360 calories, 28g carbohydrates, 25g fat, 6.7g protein.

Strawberry Banana Smoothie

Cooking time 5 min | Servings 1

Ingredients

1 ripe banana

10 oz frozen or fresh sliced strawberries

1/2 cup milk

Directions

Place all ingredients in a blender. Blend them until smooth and creamy.

Nutritional facts per serving: 303 calories, 51.73g carbohydrates, 5.88g fat, 7.97g protein.

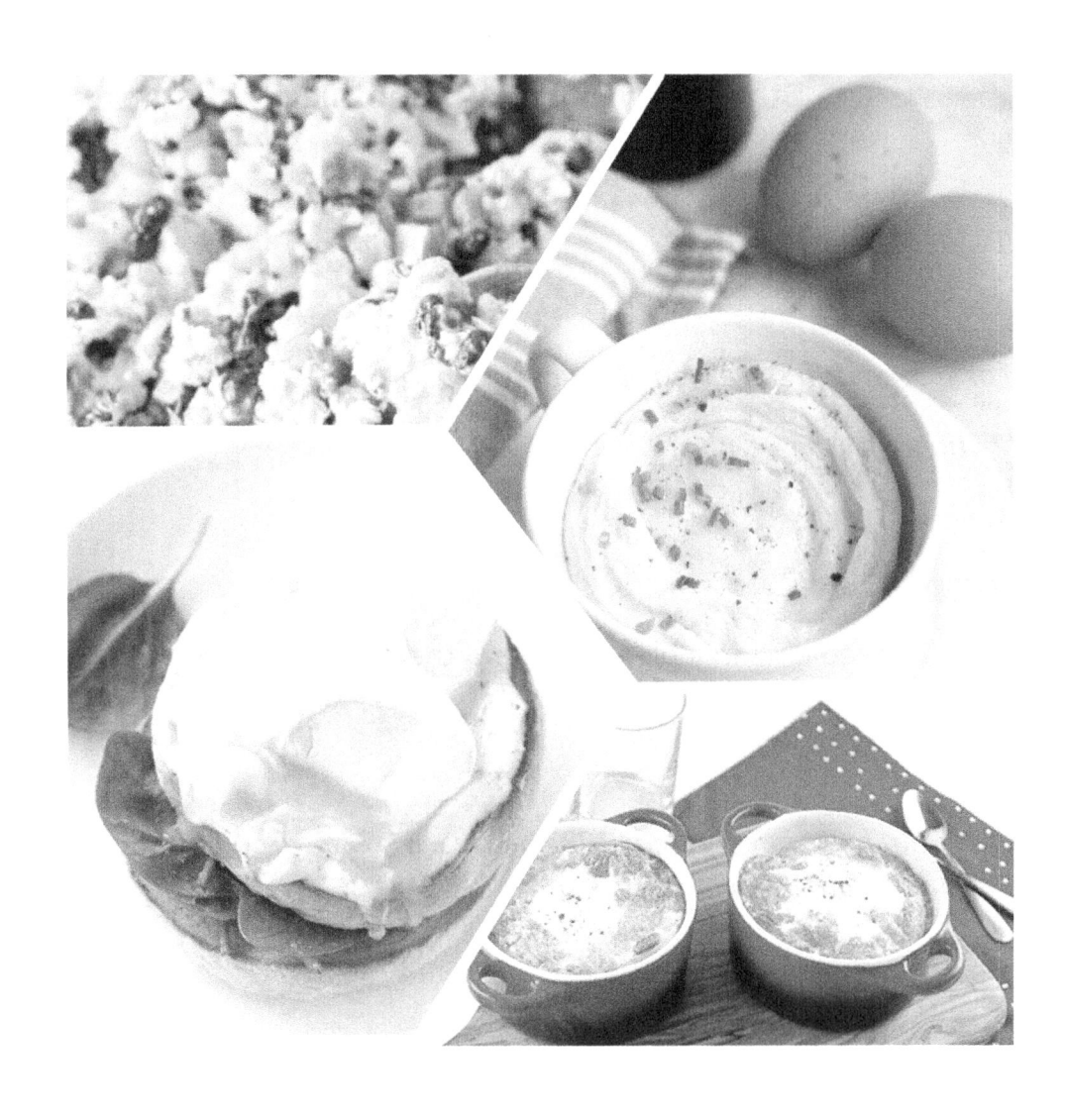

Mexican Egg Scramble

Cooking time 5 min| Servings 1

Ingredients

2 eggs

1/4 cup canned black beans

1 oz cheddar cheese, reduced-fat

2 tbsp salsa

Directions

1. Drain the beans.
2. In a medium bowl, scramble the eggs with canned beans.
3. Preheat the skillet over medium heat. Pour the mixture into the skillet. Cook stirring for 2-3 minutes.
4. Add cheddar cheese to the eggs. Cook stirring for 1 minute.
5. Remove the eggs from the skillet to the plate.
6. Top the dish with salsa.

Nutritional facts per serving: 343 calories, 10.34g carbohydrates, 21.76g fat, 24.56g protein.

1-Minute Eggs

Cooking time 2 min| Servings 1

Ingredients

1 egg

2 tbsp milk

herbs and spices, to taste

Directions

1. Beat a raw egg with milk.
2. Pour the mixture into a microwave-safe mug, and heat for 60 seconds.
3. Season with herbs or spices to taste.

Nutritional facts per serving: 111.95 calories, 2.31g carbohydrates, 7.44g fat, 8.27g protein.

Poached Eggs

Cooking time 4 min | Servings 1

Ingredients

1 egg

1 tbsp vinegar

Directions

1. Break an egg into a dish.
2. Bring a medium saucepan of water to boil; reduce heat to low.
3. Add a tablespoon of vinegar into the water. Stir the water, make a vortex.
4. Pour the egg into the center of the vortex and cook for three minutes. Make the yolk your desired doneness.

Nutritional Facts per serving: 86 calories, 0.39g carbohydrates, 6g fat, 6.99g protein.

Welsh Eggs

Cooking time 30 min | Servings 6

Ingredients

2 cups mild cheddar cheese, coarsely grated

12 eggs

Salt and seasoned pepper

Directions

1. Butter 6 ovenproof dishes lavishly. Preheat the oven to 325°F
2. Grate cheese coarsely. Sprinkle 1/4 cup of the grated cheese in the bottom of each buttered dish.
3. Break the eggs in a saucer and then slip 2eggs over the cheese's surface in each dish. Take care not to break the yolk. Allow two eggs per dish.
4. Sprinkle the remainder of the cheese over the surface of each dish. Sprinkle with salt and pepper to taste.
5. Place the dishes in the oven—Bake for 20 minutes. Serve with toasts for dipping into the egg yolk and the melted cheese.

Nutritional facts per serving: 434 calories, 0.77g carbohydrates, 33.3g fat, 29.3g protein.

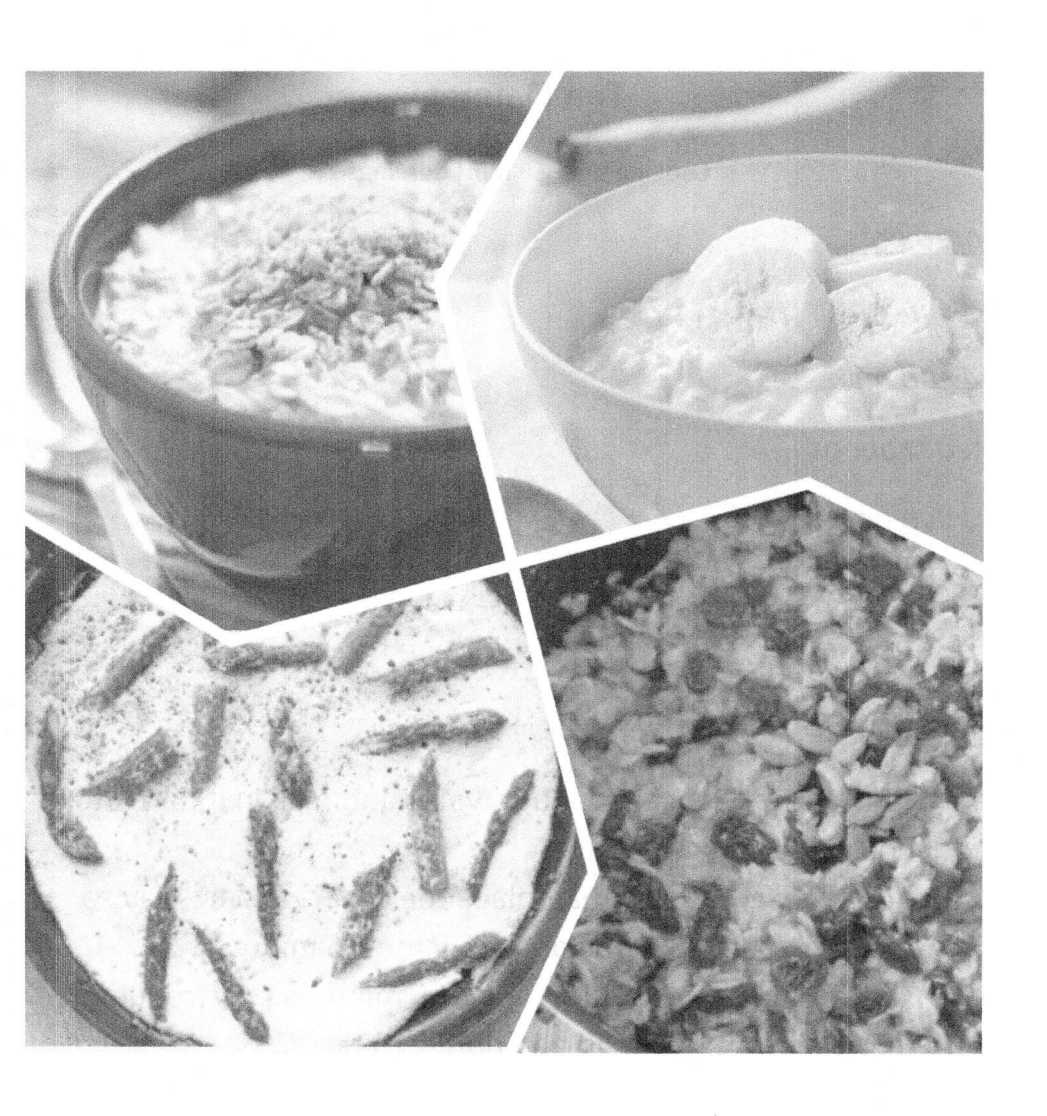

Tea Oatmeal

Cooking time 18 min| Servings 1

Ingredients

3/4 cup water

1/4 cup milk

1 tea teabags

1/2 cup oatmeal

Honey to taste

Directions

1. Take a small saucepan, pour water and milk in it. Bring to a boil.
2. Add teabag, reduce heat, place the cover on part-way so that steam can escape, and cook for 4-6 minutes.
3. Add oatmeal and cook for about 5 minutes. Stir frequently.
4. Remove from heat and add honey to taste.

Nutritional Facts per serving: 128 calories, 18g carbohydrates, 3.95g fat, 5g protein.

Tropical Oatmeal

Cooking time 6 min | Servings 1

Ingredients

1/2 cup oatmeal

1 cup water

1/2 tsp coconut extract

1/2 medium banana

Splenda sugar or sweetener (optional)

Directions

1. Cook oatmeal in the microwave or stovetop as you usually do.
2. Slice up banana, 1/4-inch slices, cut into four pieces.
3. Add coconut extract and banana to the cooked oatmeal.
4. You can add sweetener to taste.

Nutritional Facts per serving: 211 calories, 2.8g fat, 40.9g carbohydrates, 6g protein.

Egg Whites with Asparagus

Cooking time 8 min| Servings 1

Ingredients

Pam cooking spray

4 ½ oz frozen asparagus cuts

½ cup egg whites

1 tbsp parmesan cheese

Directions

1. Microwave asparagus at 100% power for 3 to 5 minutes. Place cuts into the covered microwavable baking dish with two tablespoons of water. Or use **package directions for microwaving.**
2. Drain well asparagus and separate into halves.
3. Take an 8" pan and spray it with pam. Put half the asparagus in the pan.
4. Pour egg whites over asparagus and cook for 2 minutes over medium heat.
5. Sprinkle asparagus with parmesan and broil for 4-5 minutes.

Nutritional facts per serving: 115.3 calories, 17g fat, 6.3g carbohydrate, 19.3g protein.

Oatmeal with Cardamom and Raisins

Cooking time 5 min | Servings 2

Ingredients

1 cup quick-cooking oats, raw

1 3/4 cups water

1/2 – 1 cup raisins

1/2 tsp cardamom

Directions

1. Boil water and raisins over medium heat in the saucepan.
2. Add oats to the boiling water—Cook for 1 minute. Stir often.
3. Remove the saucepan from the heat. Cover the saucepan for 3 minutes.
4. Add cardamom, mix well.
5. You can sprinkle the oat with honey or milk.

Nutritional Facts per Serving: 263.4 calories, 2.8g fat, 56.5 carbohydrates, 6.5g protein.

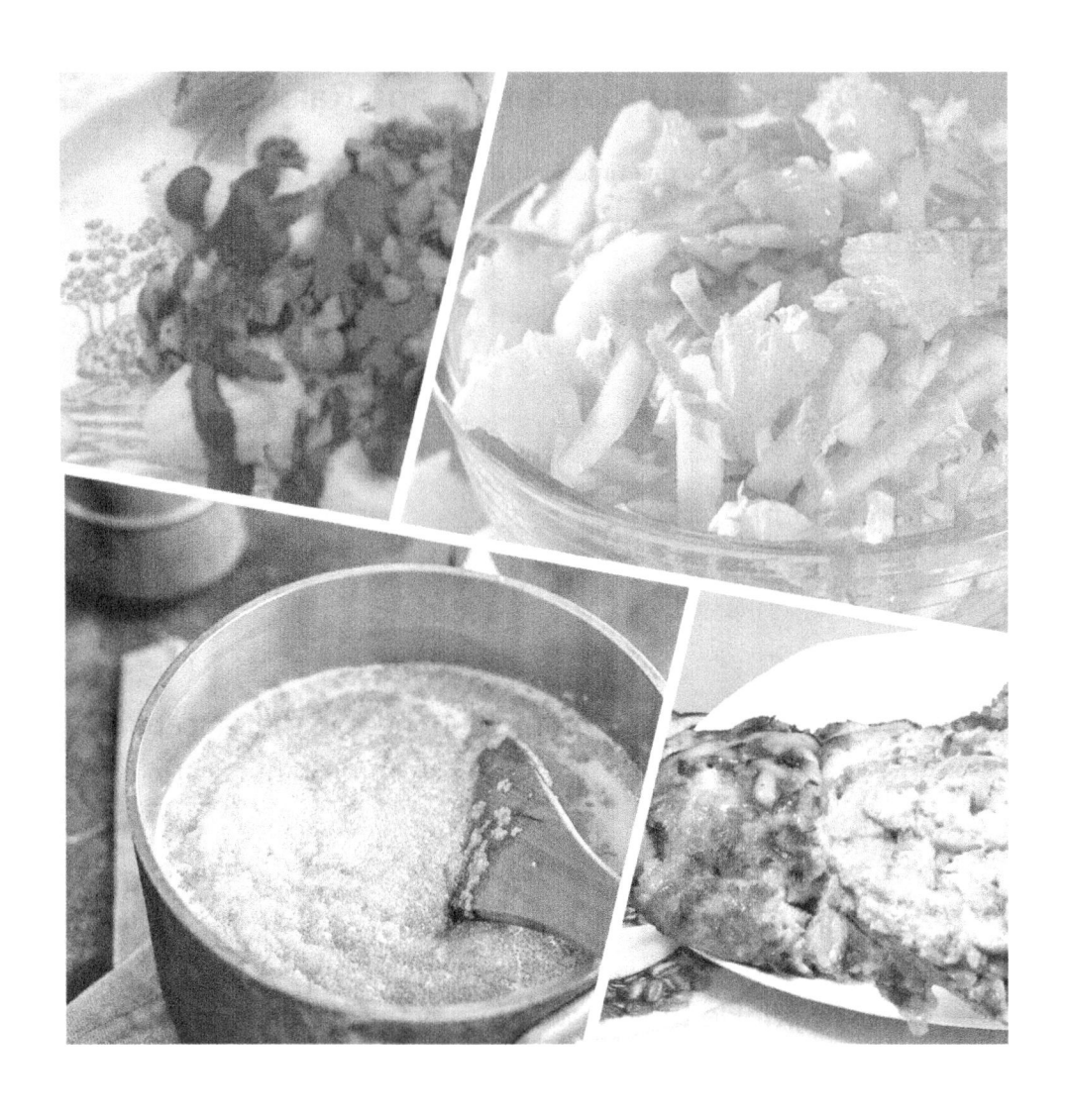

Banana Split

Cooking time 10 min| Servings 2

Ingredients

2 bananas

1/2 cup vanilla yogurt

1/4 cup raspberry jam (or strawberry)

nuts

chocolate syrup

Directions

1. Try to choose ripe and small bananas. Cut off one inch, and then slice the banana in half and place on a salad plate curving away from one another and outward.
2. Slice the small piece and place it on either side of the curved pieces.
3. Spoon whipped yogurt across the top of bananas.
4. Place jam slightly on top of yogurt.
5. Sprinkle nuts on top to taste. Use chocolate or fudge sauce.

Nutritional facts per serving: 253.6 calories, 2.4g fat, 57.4 carbohydrates, 3.6g protein.

Carrot, Apple, and Orange Salad

Cooking time 10 min| Servings 2

Ingredients

3 ½ oz carrots

3 ½ oz apples

2 oz orange

2 tbsp yogurt

1 tsp honey

Directions

1. Wash and peel the carrots. Grate finely.

2. Cut the apple into small slices.

3. Peel the orange, separate the lobes. Chop finely.

4. Stir all the ingredients in a medium bowl.

5. Mix yogurt and honey. Add the mixture to the main ingredients.

Nutritional facts per serving: 75.3 calories, 1.97g protein, 0.7g fat, 15.28g carbohydrates.

Amaranth Porridge

Cooking time 30 min | Servings 6

Ingredients

1 cup amaranth

1 small clove of garlic

1 oz onion

3 cups vegetable broth

Sea salt to taste

Directions

1. Peel the onion and garlic. Chop the onion into small cubes and chop the garlic.

2. Mix amaranth, garlic, onions, and broth in a 2.5-liter saucepan. Bring to a boil and simmer for about 20-25 minutes, until most of the liquid is absorbed. Mix well. If the resulting mixture is too liquidy or the amaranth is not completely wrinkled (it should be crunchy, but not too hard), boil slightly, stirring continuously, until thickened, about 30 seconds. Add salt.

Nutritional facts per serving: 132.5 calories, 4.8g protein, 2.42g fat, 24.71g carbohydrates.

Zucchini Omelette

Cooking time 30 min| Servings 2

Ingredients

5 tbsp fat-free cottage cheese

2 eggs + 2 egg whites

7 oz zucchini

salt

Directions

1. Beat cottage cheese with the eggs. Peel the zucchini and finely grate. Mix egg mixture and zucchini and add salt.

2. Place the mixture in a form and bake in the oven at 260 ºF for 25 minutes. Sprinkle with herbs and serve.

Nutritional facts per serving: 191 calories, 17g protein, 9.4g fat, 3.84g carbs.

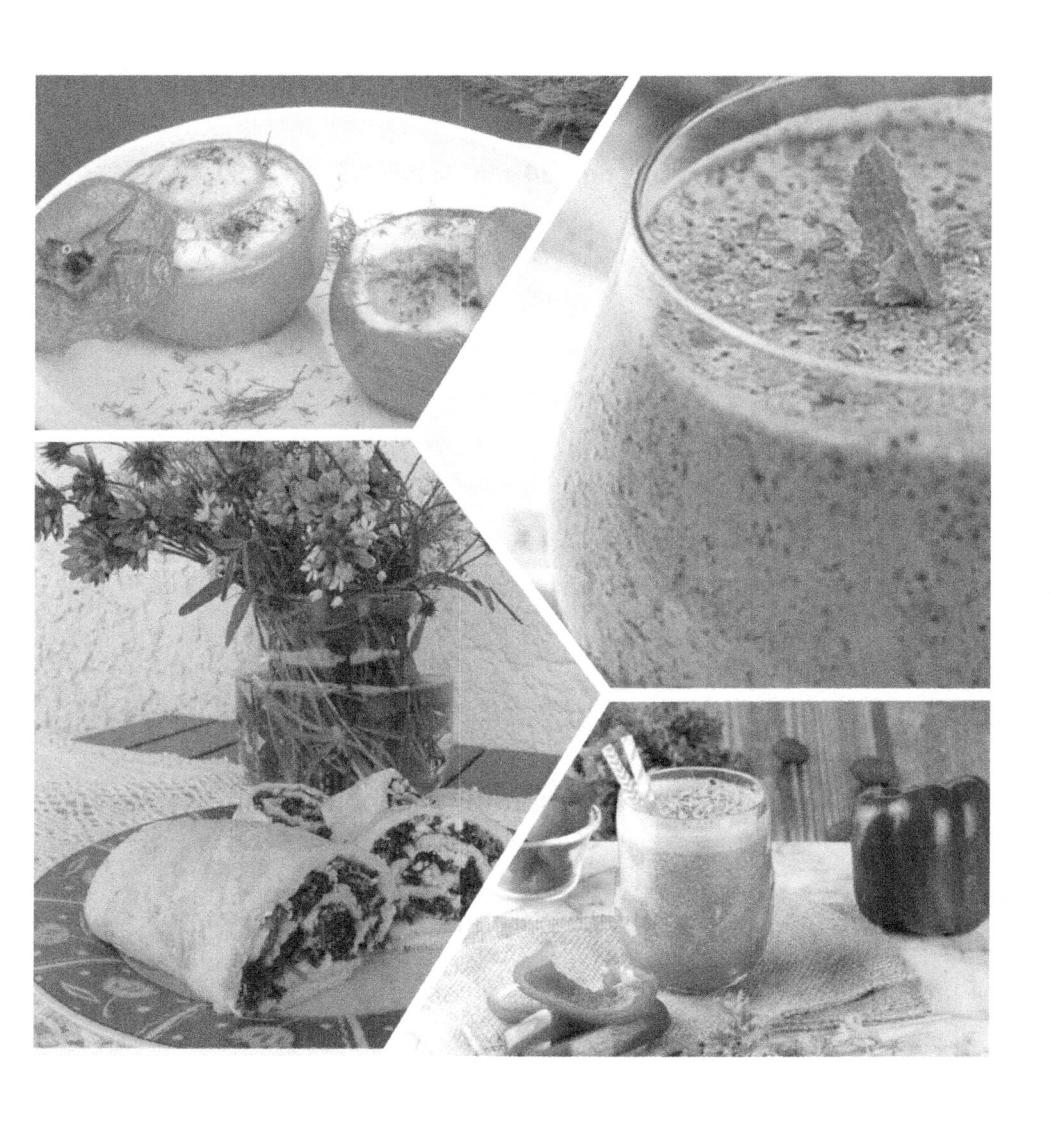

Eggs in Tomatoes

Cooking time 30 min| Servings 2

<u>*Ingredients*</u>

4 tomatoes, 2/3 lb

4 eggs

green onions to taste

salt, pepper to taste

<u>Directions</u>

1. Preheat the oven to 370 ° F.

2. Cut the caps off the tomatoes. Remove the core and seeds with a spoon.

3. Cover the baking sheet with parchment.

4. Place hollow tomatoes on a baking sheet.

5. Place an egg into each. Salt to taste.

6. Bake for 25-30 minutes.

7. Pepper to taste. Garnish with green onions.

Nutritional facts per serving: 210.7 calories, 16.06g protein, 12.37g fat, 7.8g carbohydrates.

Flax Seed Smoothie

Cooking time 10 min| Servings 1

Ingredients

3 tbsp flax seeds

2 tbsp pumpkin seeds

3 ½ oz blueberries (fresh or frozen)

3 ½ oz banana

100ml milk

Directions

1. Grind the flax and pumpkin seeds in a coffee grinder.

2. Place the berries in the blender, add ground flax and pumpkin seeds.

3. Pour milk and combine (until smoothie).

Nutritional facts per serving: 474.4 calories, 16.19g protein, 26g fat, 43.81g carbohydrates.

Roll-Up Omelet with Spinach

Cooking time 40 min | 1 serve

Ingredients

1 tsp canola oil

1 egg

1 cup baby spinach

1 tsp olive tapenade

1 tbsp crumbled goat cheese

Directions

1. Drizzle canola oil into a non-stick pan. Then, wipe with a paper towel. Heat the pan over medium heat.

2. Beat the egg and swirl it into the frying pan. Cook 2 minutes. Then, flip the egg and cook for 1 minute.

3. Carefully place the egg on a plate. In the same pan, sauté one cup of spinach for about 1 minute, until wilted.

5. Top the egg with olive tapenade and goat cheese. Then place wilted spinach on the ingredients. Roll up the egg and cut it in half.

Nutritional facts per serving: 305.22 calories, 15.5g protein, 25.27g fat, 3.51g carbohydrates.

Tomato and Bell Pepper Smoothies

Cooking time 5 min | 1 serve

Ingredients

½ cup tomato juice

½ cup carrot juice

1 bell peppers

½ tbsp lemon juice

ground black pepper

Directions

1. Wash, peel and cut peppers into medium-sized pieces. Place in a blender.

2. Add lemon juice and black ground pepper to taste. Add tomato and carrot juices. Beat.

3. Drink immediately after preparation.

Nutritional facts per serving: 89.75 calories, 4.18g protein, 0.31g fat, 18.19g carbohydrates.

Tomato and Avocado Frittata

Cooking time 10 minutes| Servings 1

Ingredients

2 eggs

½ tomato (1 oz)

¼ avocado

2 tbsp milk

1 oz greens to taste

Directions

1.   Take the eggs, beat them into a medium bowl. Add milk and whisk the ingredients well.

2.   Cut the tomato into quarters

3.   Preheat the non-stick frying pan. Put the tomato pieces on it — Cook for 1 minute.

4.   Pour egg with milk into the pan — Cook for 3-5 minutes

5.   Peel and cut the avocado into slices to your taste. Chop the greens finely.

6.   Top your frittata with avocado and greens.

Nutritional facts per serving: 324 calories, 23.16g fat, 17.69g protein, 9.08g carbohydrate

LUNCH AND DINNER

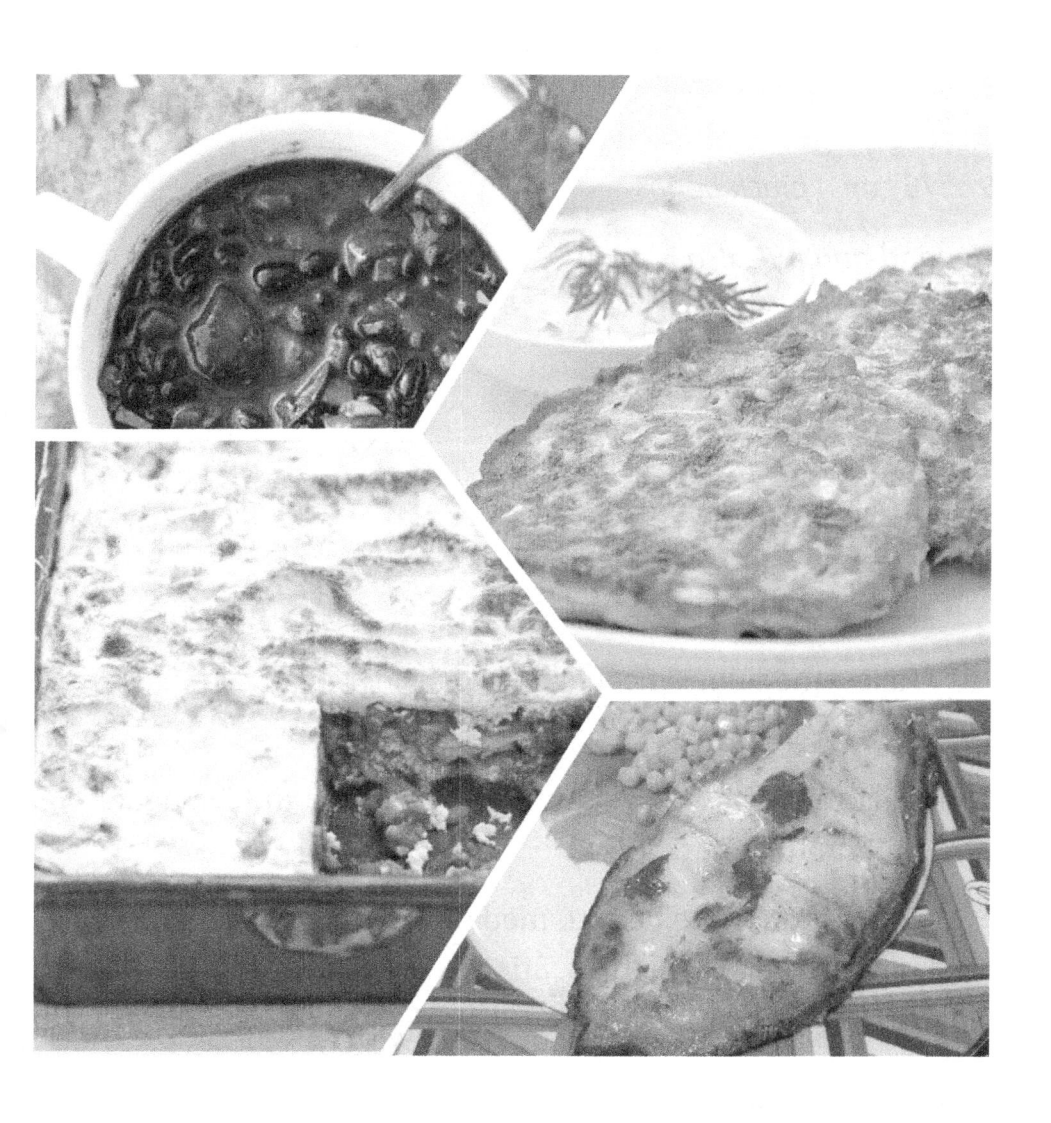

Black Bean Soup

Cooking time 20 min | Servings 4

Ingredients

45 oz (3 cans) black beans

1 lb good-quality salsa

½ cup fresh cilantro

2 tsp cumin, ground

1 clove garlic

Directions

1. Mince the garlic.

2. Take a medium saucepan, place all ingredients in it. Beans must be with the liquid.

3. Heat the beans with the spices over medium-high heat. Cook until simmering.

4. Then, reduce the heat to medium-low. Cover the saucepan and simmer for 10-12 minutes. Stir the beans.

5. Chop cilantro for serving the soup with it.

Nutritional facts per serving: 319 calories, 21.7g protein, 1g fat, 55.5g carbohydrates.

Lentil Lasagne

Cooking time 60 min| Servings 4

Ingredients

1 package no-pre lasagne sheets

2 ½ cups creamy tomato soup

1 cup pre-cooked lentils

6 ½ oz green pesto

2 handfuls cheese

Directions

1. Preheat the oven to 350 F.

2. Take the pan, pour a part of the soup on the bottom of it. Place the first layer of lasagna sheets. Then pour a portion of tomato soup, top it with the lentils and pesto. Then repeat.

3. Finish the lasagna with the topping of the rest of the tomato soup and sprinkle with cheese, last dollops of pesto.

4. Cover the pan, bake for 50 minutes.

Nutritional facts per serving: 546 calories, 18.4g protein, 1g fat, 49.9g carbohydrates.

Zucchini Fritters

Cooking time 25 min | Servings 14

Ingredients

4 cups shredded zucchini

2/3 cup flour, all-purpose

2 eggs

1/3 cup scallions

2 tbsp olive oil

Directions

1. Shred the zucchini. Take the colander, set it over the bowl, and place the vegetable in it. Sprinkle the zucchini with salt lightly. Leave for 10 minutes.

2. Squeeze out as much liquid as possible from the zucchini with your hands.

3. Transfer the main ingredient to the large bowl, add flour, eggs, scallions, salt (to your taste). Stir the ingredients well.

4. Take the plate and line it with paper towels.

5. Preheat the saute pan over medium heat, add oil.

6. Scoop three tablespoons of mixture in hot oil. Press the mixture into round lightly, at least 2 inches apart.

7. Cook the pancakes for 2-3 minutes, flip once and cook an additional 2 minutes, cook until golden.

8. Transfer the zucchini fritters to the paper towel-lined plate, sprinkle them with salt immediately.

9. Top the pancakes with sour cream (optional).

Nutritional Facts per Serving: 110 calories, 4g protein, 6g fat, 12g carbohydrates.

Roasted Corn and Tilapia

Cooking time 20 min| Servings 4

Ingredients

¼ cup plain yogurt

2 tsp chili powder

¼ tsp salt

4 tilapia filets or you can choose other mild white fish

1 ½ cups corn (fresh or frozen)

1 wedge lime or lemon

Directions

1. Preheat the grill to high.
2. At the same time, take a small bowl. Pour yogurt, salt, and chili in it, combine well.
3. Take a large baking dish for four pieces of tilapia. Spread a thin layer of sauce over the bottom of the baking dish.
4. Place the fish on top of the sauce. Then pour the remaining sauce on the fish.
5. Top the fish with the corn.
6. Cook the fish for about 10 minutes. The corn must be slightly charred and fish through cooked.

7. Serve the dish with lime or lemon.

Nutritional facts per serving: 333.7 calories, 64.1g protein, 5.9g fat, 7.1g carbohydrates

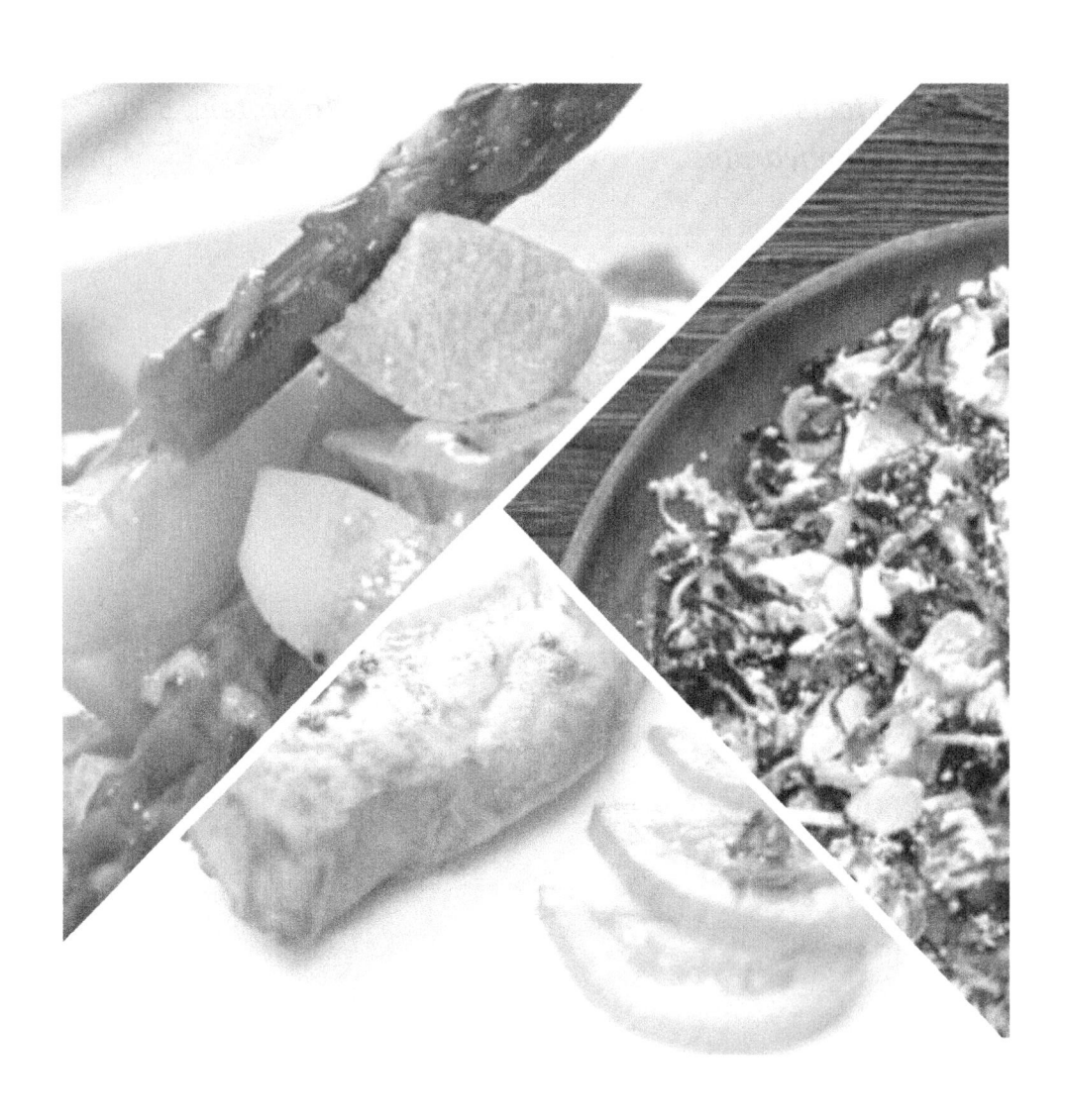

Buttermilk Chicken

Cooking time 8 h 20 min | Servings 12

Ingredients

12 chicken breasts (boneless and skinless)

1 ½ cups buttermilk

4 thyme sprigs

4 garlic cloves

½ tsp salt

Directions

1. Take a large bowl and pour buttermilk; place thyme, garlic, salt in it. Combine all ingredients well.

2. Add chicken to the mixture, coat with the sauce well. Refrigerate for 8 hours and turn occasionally.

3. Drain chicken, discard marinade.

4. Grill the chicken over medium heat for 7-10 minutes per side.

Nutritional facts per serving: 189 calories, 35g protein, 4g fat, 1g carbohydrates.

Shredded Kale and Brussels Sprouts Salad

Cooking time 15 min | Servings 6

Ingredients

8 oz kale

½ lb Brussels sprouts

½ cup pistachios

½ cup honey-mustard salad dressing

¼ cup shredded Parmesan cheese

Directions

1. Slice the kale and Brussels sprouts thinly, chop pistachios coarsely.

2. Take a large bowl, place all ingredients in it, combine the mixture well.

Nutritional facts per serving: 207 calories, 14g protein, 7g fat, 16g carbohydrates.

Nicoise Salad with Asparagus

Cooking time 20 min | Servings 4

Ingredients

1 lb red potatoes, small

1 lb asparagus

7 ½ oz boiled tuna

½ cup pitted Greek olives

½ cup zesty Italian dressing

Directions

1. Take a large saucepan, pour water in it, place the potatoes. Bring water to a boil.

2. Reduce heat, cook until tender for about 12 minutes. Add asparagus during the last 3 minutes of cooking.

3. Drain asparagus and potatoes after cooking and drop the vegetables into ice water.

4. Take four plates, divide asparagus and potatoes, add boiled tuna and halved olives. Sprinkle with dressing.

Nutritional facts per serving: 260 calories, 16.8g protein, 18.7g fat, 29.3g carbohydrates.

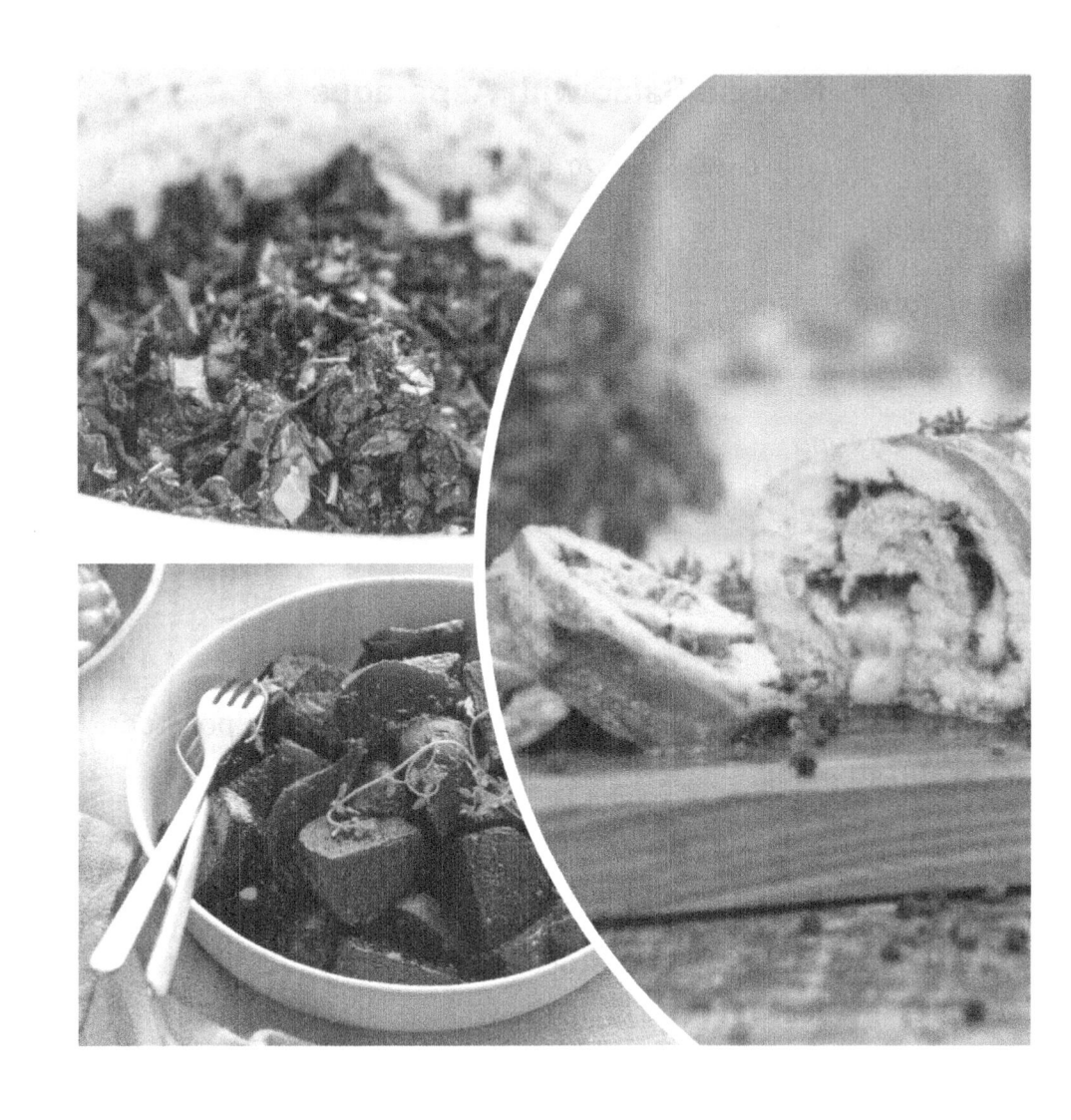

Warm Garlic Greens

Cooking time 30 min| Servings 4

Ingredients

1 lb kale

5 garlic cloves

2 tbsp olive oil

¼ tsp salt

¼ cup chopped oil-packed sun-dried tomatoes

Directions

1. Trim and torn kale, mince garlic, chop tomatoes. Pour the water into a medium stockpot, bring to a boil. Place kale in it, cover, and cook for 15 minutes, until tender.

3. Take a slotted spoon and remove the kale from the water. Discard the water.

4. Pour the oil into the same pot, heat over medium heat. Place tomatoes, garlic in it, cook for 1 minute.

5. Add kale, salt, and cook for 5 minutes, stirring.

Nutritional facts per serving: 137 calories, 4g protein, 9g fat, 14g carbohydrates.

Chicken Pesto Roll-Ups

Cooking time 45 min| Servings 4

Ingredients

4 boneless skinless chicken breast halves

1/2 cup prepared pesto, divided

1 lb medium fresh mushrooms, sliced

4 slices reduced-fat provolone cheese, halved

Directions

1. Preheat the oven to 350°F.

2. Take the chicken breasts and pound them with a meat mallet to 1/4-in thickness.

3. Spread 1/4 cup pesto over chicken breasts.

4. Coarsely chop half of the sliced mushrooms. Scatter remaining sliced mushrooms in a 15x10x1-in.

5. Baking pan coated with cooking spray. Top each chicken breast with a fourth of the chopped mushrooms and a halved cheese slice. Roll up chicken from a short side; secure with toothpicks. Place seam side down on top of the sliced mushrooms.

6. Bake for about 25-30 minutes.

7.   Preheat broiler. Top chicken with remaining pesto and cheese. Broil until cheese is melted and browned, 3-5 minutes longer. Discard toothpicks.

Nutritional facts per serving: 374 calories, 44g protein, 17g fat, 7g carbohydrates.

Roasted Beet Wedges

Cooking time 1 h 15 min | Servings 4

Ingredients

1 lb beets

4 tsp olive oil

½ tsp kosher salt

4 fresh rosemary sprigs

Directions

1. Peel the beets and cut each into six wedges.

2. At the same time, preheat the oven to 400°F.

3. Place the beets' pieces in the bowl, add olive oil, salt, combine gently.

4. Place a piece of foil in a baking pan, arrange beets on foil, top with rosemary, fold foil around beets, and seal tightly.

5. Bake the beets until tender for 1 hour; after cooking, discard rosemary sprigs.

Nutritional facts per serving: 92 calories, 2g protein, 5g fat, 12g carbohydrate.

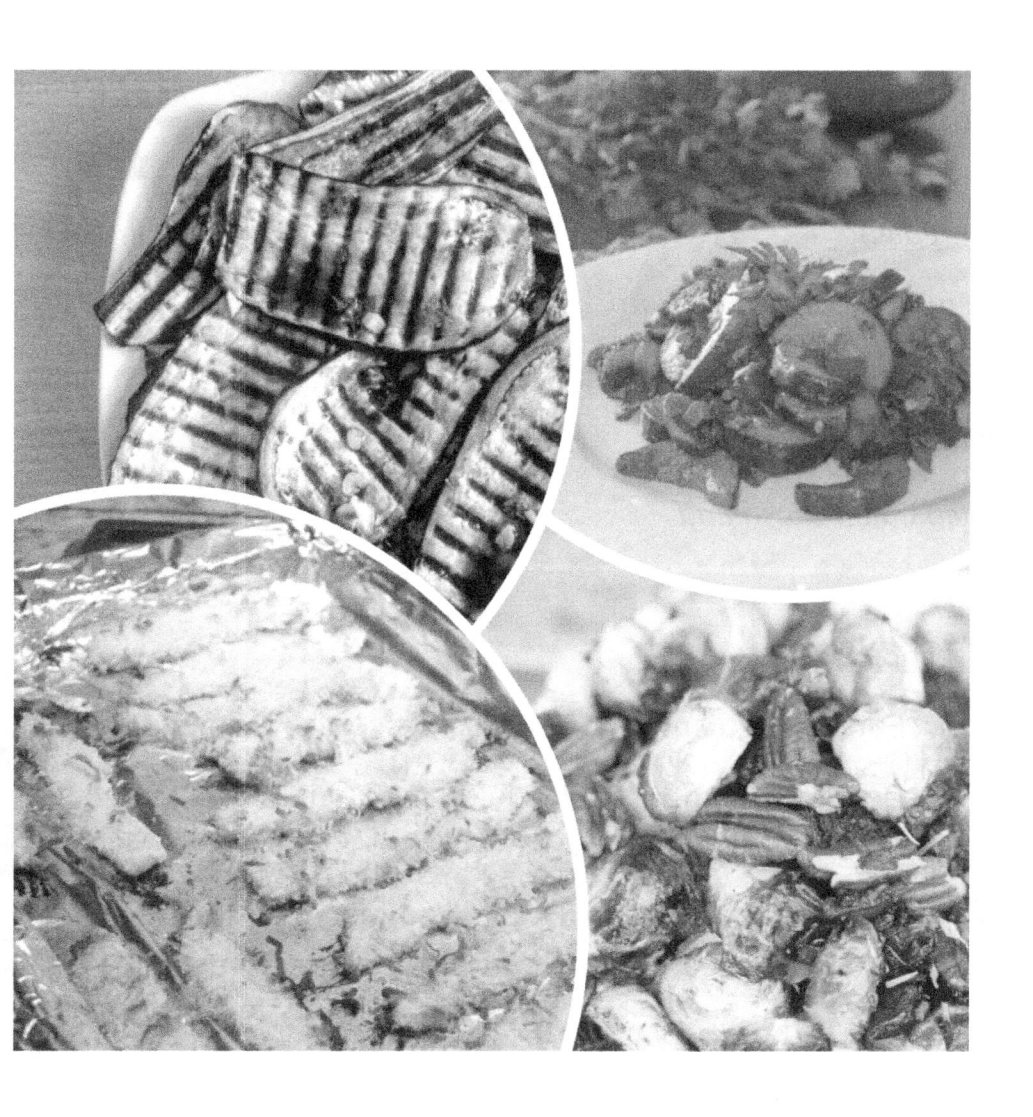

Grilled Eggplant

Cooking time 20 min | Servings 8

Ingredients

2 small eggplants, cut into 1/2-inch slices

¼ cup olive oil

2 tbsp lime juice

3 tsp Cajun seasoning

Directions

1. Cut the eggplants into ½-inch slices, brush them with oil.

2. Drizzle eggplant with lime juice and Cajun seasoning. Let stand for 5 minutes.

3. Grill eggplant over medium heat until tender for 10 minutes, 4-5 minutes per side. You can broil the eggplant too.

Nutritional facts per serving: 88 calories, 1g protein, 7g fat, 7g carbohydrate.

Braised Beef and Zucchini

Cooking time 1 h 30 min | Servings 1

Ingredients

1/3 lb beef

3 oz zucchini

½ onion

1 tbsp olive oil

Salt and pepper to taste

Directions

1. Cut beef and onions into small pieces.

2. Put the olive oil in a frying pan and add the meat and onions. Fry until golden brown on high heat.

3. Add a little water, cover, and stew for one hour on low heat.

4. Cut the zucchini into slices. Add the vegetables and spices to the beef and stew for 30 minutes.

Nutritional facts per serving: 403 calories, 30.38g protein, 28.78g fat, 7g carbohydrate.

Coconut Chicken Strips

Cooking time 35 min | Servings 4

Ingredients

1 lb boneless skinless chicken breasts

2 tbsp extra virgin olive oil

¼ tsp pepper

½ tsp salt

1 cup unsweetened coconut flakes (or use shredded coconut)

Directions

1. Preheat the oven to 390 ºF.

2. Slice the chicken into strips. Coat the chicken with olive oil.

3. Mix salt, pepper, and coconut in a bowl. Cover chicken with the mixture.

4. Place the chicken strips on the baking sheet. Bake for 30 minutes, until golden brown.

5. Serve the chicken with the sauce.

Nutritional facts per serving: 515 calories, 32g protein, 38.8g fat, 7g carbohydrate.

Pecan Butter with Brussels Sprouts

Cooking time 30 min| Servings 1

Ingredients

1 cup Brussels sprouts

1/8 cup chopped pecans

½ tbsp Earth Balance (dairy-free butter)

½ tsp brown sugar

¼ tsp lemon juice

Salt to taste

Directions

1. Trim off bottoms of Brussels sprouts. Cut "X" in the depths.
2. Boil water in a large pot. Add salt.
3. Boil Brussels sprouts for 10 minutes. Drain and place into ice bath sprouts. Cut them in half.
4. Heat Earth Balance over medium heat.
5. Add chopped pecans, cook for 2 minutes.
6. Place the sprouts on the frying pan. Cook over medium-high heat until browned. Brown the other side too.
7. Add sugar, lemon juice, salt. Combine the ingredients.

8. Place Brussels on a serving dish. Top them with browned pecans.

Nutritional facts per serving: 284.16 calories, 12g protein, 18.8g fat, 21.97g carbohydrate

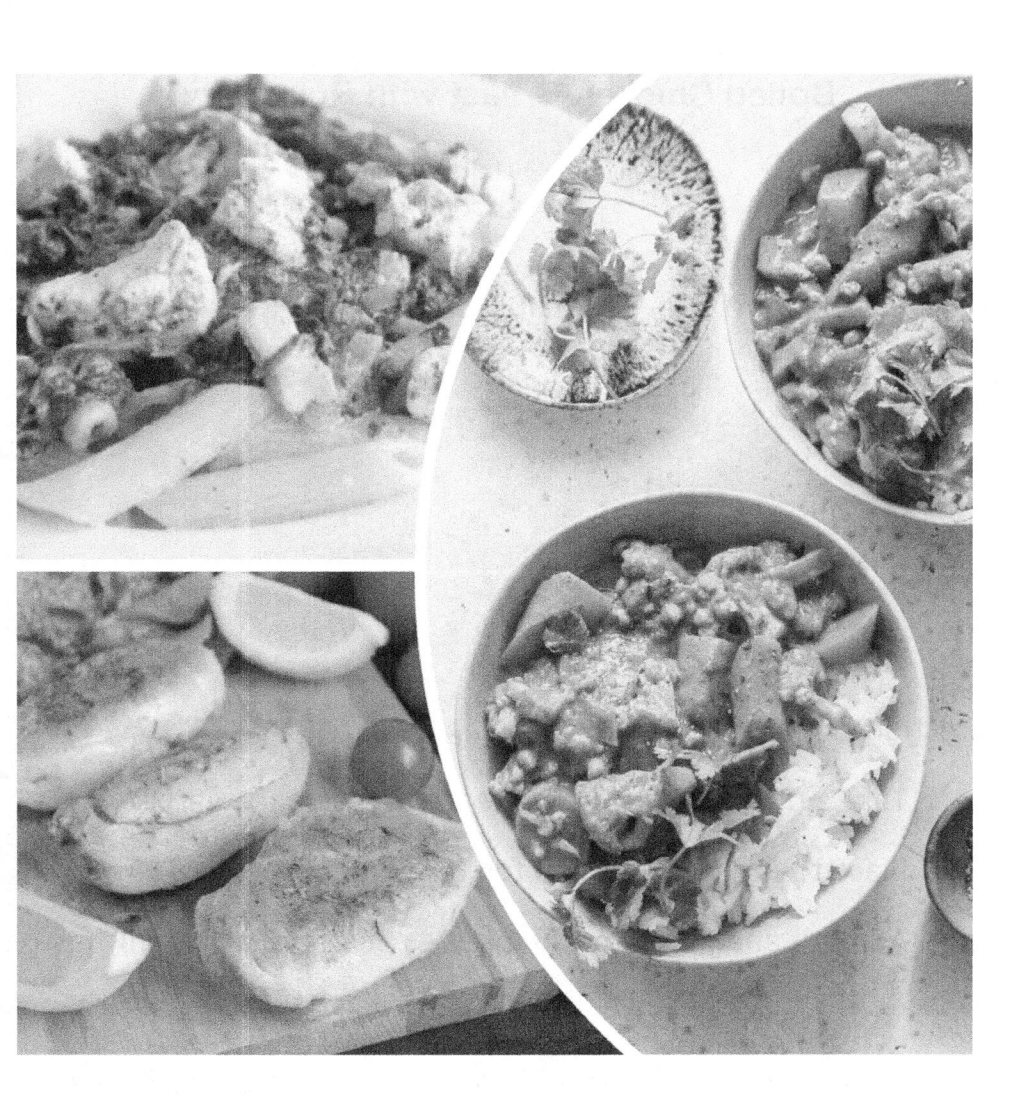

Boiled Chicken Breast with Rosemary

Cooking time 30 min | Servings 1

Ingredients

6 oz chicken breast boneless, skinless

rosemary

clove of garlic

salt and pepper to taste

1000 ml water

Directions

1. Take a pan, pour it with water. Add rosemary, garlic.
2. Place the breast in it. Boil for 15-20 min.
3. Add salt and pepper for 5 minutes before cooking finishes.

Nutritional facts per serving: 226 calories, 47.2g protein, 3.8g fat, 0.8g carbohydrate

Salmon Spinach Pasta

Cooking time 20 min| Servings 2

Ingredients

½ lb penne

2 skinless salmon fillets

2 oz sundried tomatoes

3 oz bag spinach

Directions

1. Cook the pasta according to instructions on the pack.

2. Take and preheat the frying pan, pour tomato's oil in it. Add tomatoes, cook for 4 minutes.

3. Place the fish in the pan. After that, add cooked pasta, spinach, stir for 2-3 minutes.

Nutritional facts per serving: 300 calories, 41.2g protein, 12g fat, 2g carbohydrate

Chicken & Celery Root Tikka Masala

Cooking time 35 min| Servings 4

Ingredients

2 tbsp canola oil

2 cups peeled celery root

1 ¼ lb boneless, skinless chicken thighs

1 12-oz jar Tikka Masala simmer sauce

1 cup frozen peas

Directions

1. At first, you have to thaw the peas.

2. And let's start to prepare for cooking. Take the celery root, peel, and dice it: Trim and cut chicken.

3. Take a large non-stick skillet, heat one tablespoon of oil in it over medium-high heat.

4. Add celery to the skillet, cook, and occasionally stir for about 5 minutes. Cook until brown.

5. Add another tablespoon of oil, chicken—Cook for about 4 minutes.

6. After that, add sauce, combine all ingredients gently. Cook for 10 minutes until the celery tendering and chicken cooked through.

7. Add peas, stir and simmer for 1 minute.

Nutritional facts per serving: 437 calories, 31.4g protein, 12g fat, 18.5g carbohydrate

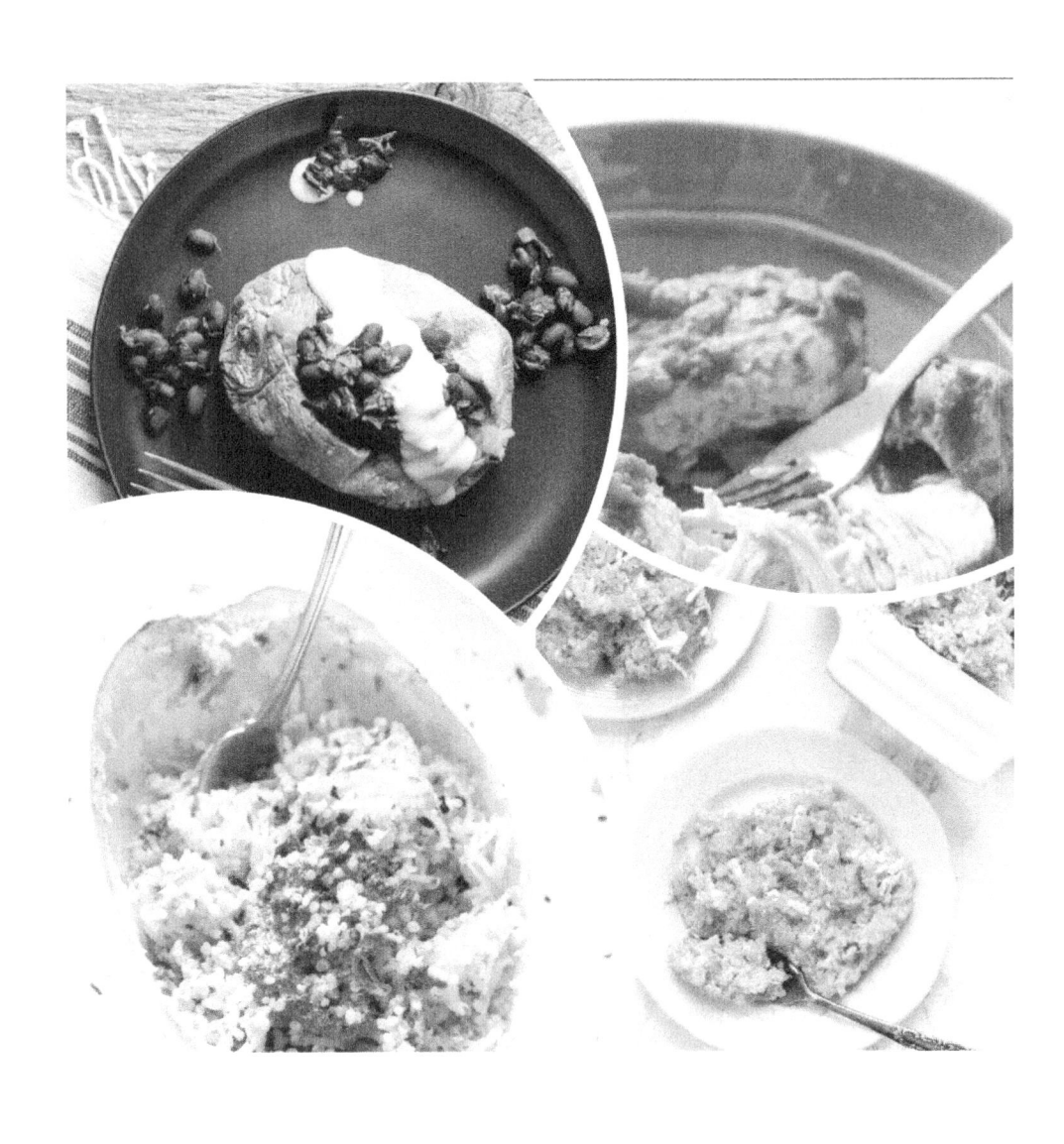

Stuffed Potato and Hummus Dressing

Cooking time 35 min| Servings 1

<u>Ingredients</u>

1 large sweet potato, scrubbed

¾ cup chopped kale

1 cup canned black beans, rinsed

¼ cup hummus

2 tbsp water

<u>Directions</u>

1. Clean sweet potatoes, take the fork and prick the potatoes all over. Microwave the vegetables until cooked. It will take you 10 minutes on "High."

2. Wash the kale, drain. Slice it. Take the medium saucepan and place the kale in it, cover the pot, cook, and stir once or twice. The kale must be wilted.

3. Add the beans, water. Uncover the saucepan, cook stirring occasionally. The mixture must be steaming hot.

5. Split the potatoes open, top the kale mixture. Garnish the meal with hummus.

Nutritional facts per serving: 472 calories, 21.1g protein, 7g fat, 85.3g carbohydrate

Chicken Fillet with Salsa Sauce.

Cooking time 45 min | Servings 2

Ingredients

1 lb boneless chicken breast

1/2 tsp salt

3/4 tsp cumin

a pinch of oregano

1 cup salsa sauce

Directions

1. Place the chicken fillets into the medium bowl. Rub the spices into the chicken.

2. Place the chicken into the pot, cover it with sauce, and cook for 40 minutes until the chicken is done.

Nutritional facts per serving: 315 calories, 60g protein, 3.5g fat, 1g carbohydrate

Squash Boats with Pesto Spaghetti

Cooking time 45 min | Servings 2

Ingredients

1 medium spaghetti squash

1 tbsp olive oil

1/3 cup pesto

1/4 cup quinoa

Salt, pepper, and chili flakes to garnish

Directions

1. Preheat the oven to 400ºF.

2. Take the spaghetti squash and slice it in half lengthwise. Scoop out the seeds.

3. Boil the quinoa.

4. Drizzle the halves of the squash with oil and salt-pepper mixture.

5. Take the baking sheet and place the squash pieces with the oiled side facing up. Roast the squash for 40 minutes. You must shred it with a fork.

6. After roasting, remove the squash from the oven, cool for a few minutes.

7. Scrape the inside of the squash pieces, and you will get the "noodles." Tops the squash with pesto, boiled quinoa.

8. You can use red pepper flakes for garnishing.

Nutritional facts per serving: 409 calories, 7g protein, 22g fat, 49g carbohydrates

5-Ingredient Quinoa Mac and Cheese

Cooking time 40 min| Servings 6

Ingredients

4 cups cubed butternut squash

1/4 cup almond milk

1/4 cup nutritional yeast or parmesan

4 cups cooked quinoa

1 cup shredded vegan cheese or shredded cheese of choice

Directions

1. Preheat oven to 375 F.

2. Peel, seed, and cube the butternut squash. Chop into 1" chunks. Take a stockpot, cover with 1" of water, cook for about 15 minutes. After cooking, drain, and transfer to a blender squash.

4. Pour almond milk, add nutritional yeast into the blender. Blend on "High." It would help if you got a silky smooth and creamy mixture.

5. Transfer squash mixture to a bowl, add quinoa, cheese to the bowl. Combine all ingredients well.

6. Choose a baking dish, place the mixture into it. Bake for 30 minutes, until bubbly.

Nutritional facts per serving: 259 calories, 7g protein, 6g fat, 42g carbohydrates

Stuffed Bell Pepper with Tomato and Chicken

Cooking time 1 hour 10 min. | Servings 4 (8 halves)

Ingredients

4 bell papers

1 lb chicken breast

5 oz tomato

2 oz parmesan cheese

2 tbsp Greek yogurt

Salt, pepper, onion, or garlic to taste

Directions

1. Preheat the oven to 350 °F. Lean the baking sheet with parchment.

2. Wash and chop chicken finely. Place the fillet into the mixing bowl.

3. Cut the tomatoes into small cubes too. Add them to the chicken.

4. Grate Parmesan finely. Add to the chicken mixture. Combine all ingredients gently.

5. Wash and cut the bell pepper into halves. Remove the seeds.

6. Fill the pepper with a chicken-tomato mixture. Place stuffed pepper on the baking sheet. Bake for 40-50 minutes

Nutritional facts per serving: 245 calories, 23.16g fat, 6.8g protein, 9.96g carbohydrate

DESSERTS

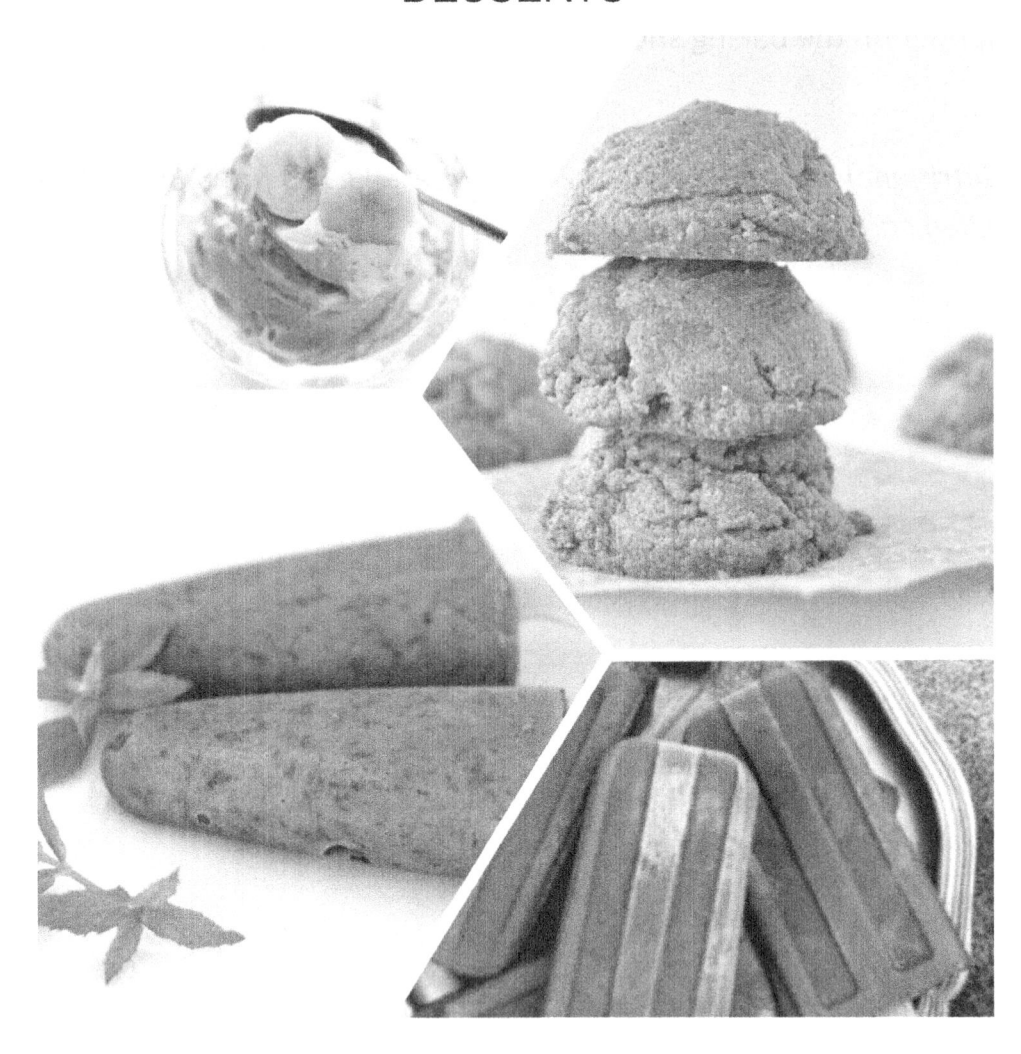

Flourless Chocolate Cookies

Cooking time 15 min | Servings 9 cookies

Ingredients

1 cup nut butter or almond

1/4 cup and 1 teaspoon maple syrup

1 tsp cacao powder

1/4 tsp baking powder

You can add sea salt, chocolate chips, shredded coconut

Directions

1. Preheat the oven to 350 °F.

2. Place all ingredients in a food processor, combine them well. You will get the dough. Form the balls.

3. Lined a baking sheet with parchment paper, place the balls onto it.

4. Bake for 10 minutes.

5. Let completely cool before removing from the sheet.

Nutritional facts per serving (per cookie): 200 calories, 0.24g protein, 20.3g fat, 4.1g carbohydrates

Banana Ice Cream

Cooking time 2 hours | Servings 1

Ingredients

2 peeled and frozen bananas

2 tsp almond butter

2 tbsp almond milk

You can add nuts, chocolate chips, fruit, coconut to your taste.

Directions

1. Cut peeled and frozen bananas into chunks.

2. Mix the bananas and the milk in a food processor.

3. Add nut butter to the partly chopped bananas. Combine all ingredients well. You will get a soft-serve consistency.

4. If you want to add nuts, chocolate chips, fruits, or coconut flakes to the banana mixture, combine gently.

5. Pour the mixture into the container and freeze for about 60-90 minutes.

Nutritional facts per serving (per cookie): 168.24 calories, 1.44g protein, 17.4g fat, 2. 24g carbohydrates

Berries and Cream Popsicles

Cooking time 2 h 5 min| Servings 6 popsicles

Ingredients

1 can full-fat coconut milk, unsweetened

1 1/2 cups blueberries

3 tbsp maple syrup

Directions

1. Pour all ingredients into the food processor. Blend for about 90 seconds.

2. Pour the mixture into popsicle molds or smoothie pop molds.

3. Place the molds into the refrigerator for 2 hours

Nutritional facts per serving (per cookie): 149 calories, 1.75g protein, 10.1g fat, 12. 34g carbohydrates.

Vegan Fudgsicles

Cooking time 2 hours | Servings 5 fudgesicles

Ingredients

1 can full-fat coconut milk

1/2 cup cocoa powder

1/4 cup maple syrup

Directions

1. Pour all ingredients into a food processor. Mix for about 1 minute.

2. Pour this coconut mixture into ice cream pop molds. Put the molds in the freezer for about 2 hours.

Nutritional facts per serving (per fudgesicle): 185 calories, 5.2g protein, 12.8g fat, 12.7g carbohydrates.

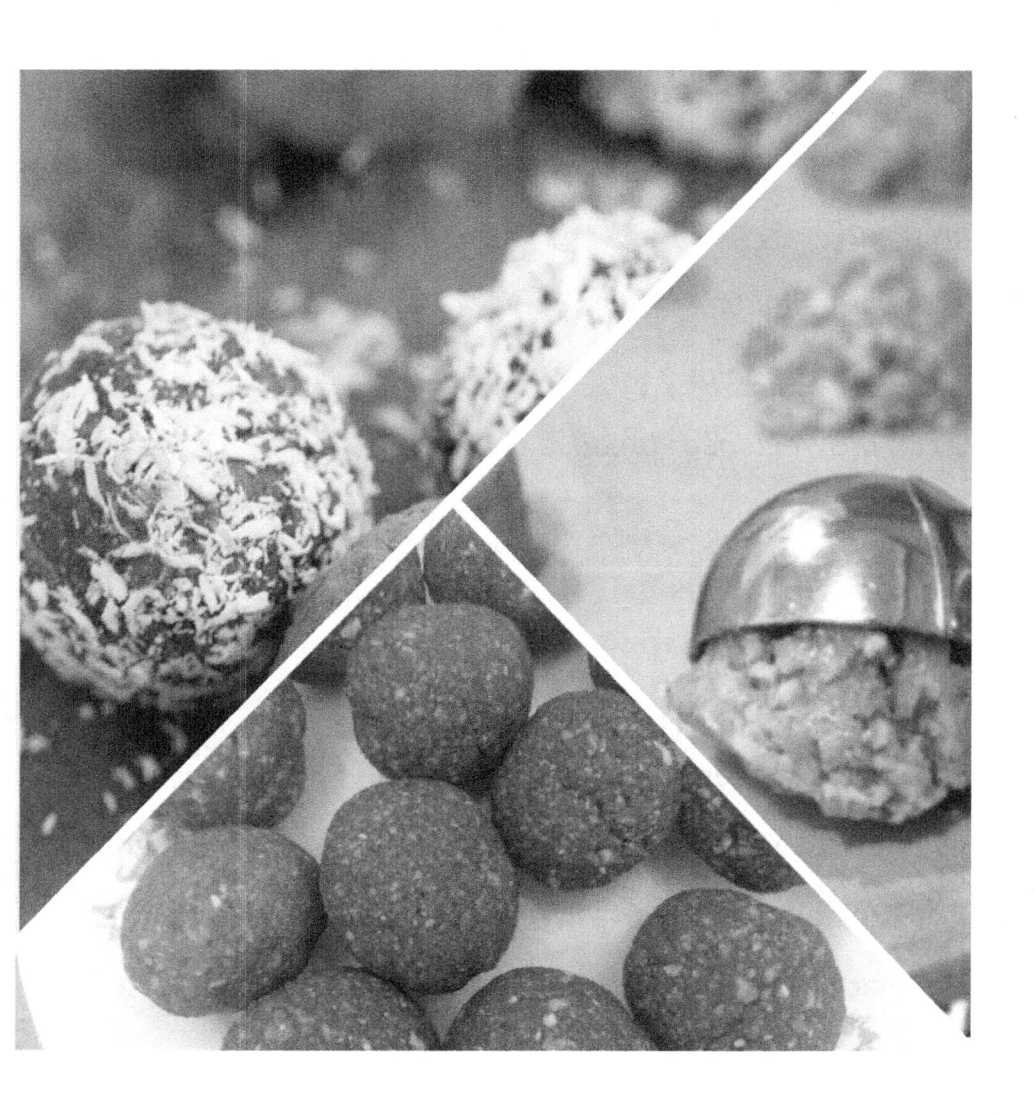

Peanuts Coconuts Bites

Cooking time 10 min | Servings 10 bites

Ingredients

1 1/2 cups peanuts

1 cup chocolate chips

1/2 cup unsweetened shredded coconut

3 tbsp water

Directions

1. Place peanuts, chocolate chips, shredded coconut into the food processor, blend for a minute or two.
2. Add the water slowly and pulse until the sticky dough.
3. The dough will look a little loose, but you can form the balls.
4. Place the balls into the refrigerator.

Nutritional facts per serving (per fudgesicle): 364 calories, 10.2g protein, 27.1g fat, 15.6g carbohydrates.

Chocolate Bites

Cooking time 5 min| Servings 6 bites

Ingredients

12 dates

1/2 cup unsweetened shredded coconut

Pinch a sea salt

1/4 cup cocoa powder

2 tbsp coconut oil

Directions

1. Pit the dates, and soak them in water for 30 minutes. Drain the water and place the dates in a food processor. Add the coconut there too, and you can add one tablespoon of water to the dates. Blend for 1 minute or less.

3. Make the balls forming the dough with your hands or a cookie scoop. Place the balls on a lined baking sheet. Place the sheet into the freezer for at least 30 minutes.

5. Take a small bowl, place the cocoa powder and coconut oil in it. Whisk the ingredients until smooth.

6. Take a spoon, and drizzle a little onto the tops of each bite. Stick back into the freezer.

Nutritional facts per serving (per bite): 199 calories, 3g protein, 13.7g fat, 16.4g carbohydrates.

Cinnamon Pecan Cookies

Cooking time 15 min| Servings 10 cookies

Ingredients

2 cups raw pecans

1 1/2 tsp cinnamon

10 dates

1/2 tsp sea salt to taste

Directions

1. Preheat oven to 350 °F.

2. Pit the dates and soak them for 15 minutes. Drain the water.

3. Place all ingredients in a food processor, combine them, and mix until formed dough.

4. Make the balls forming the dough with your hands or a cookie scoop.

5. Place the balls on the lined baking sheet—Bake for 10 minutes.

Nutritional Facts per Serving (per cookie): 303 calories, 4g protein, 28.8g fat, 8.7g carbohydrates.

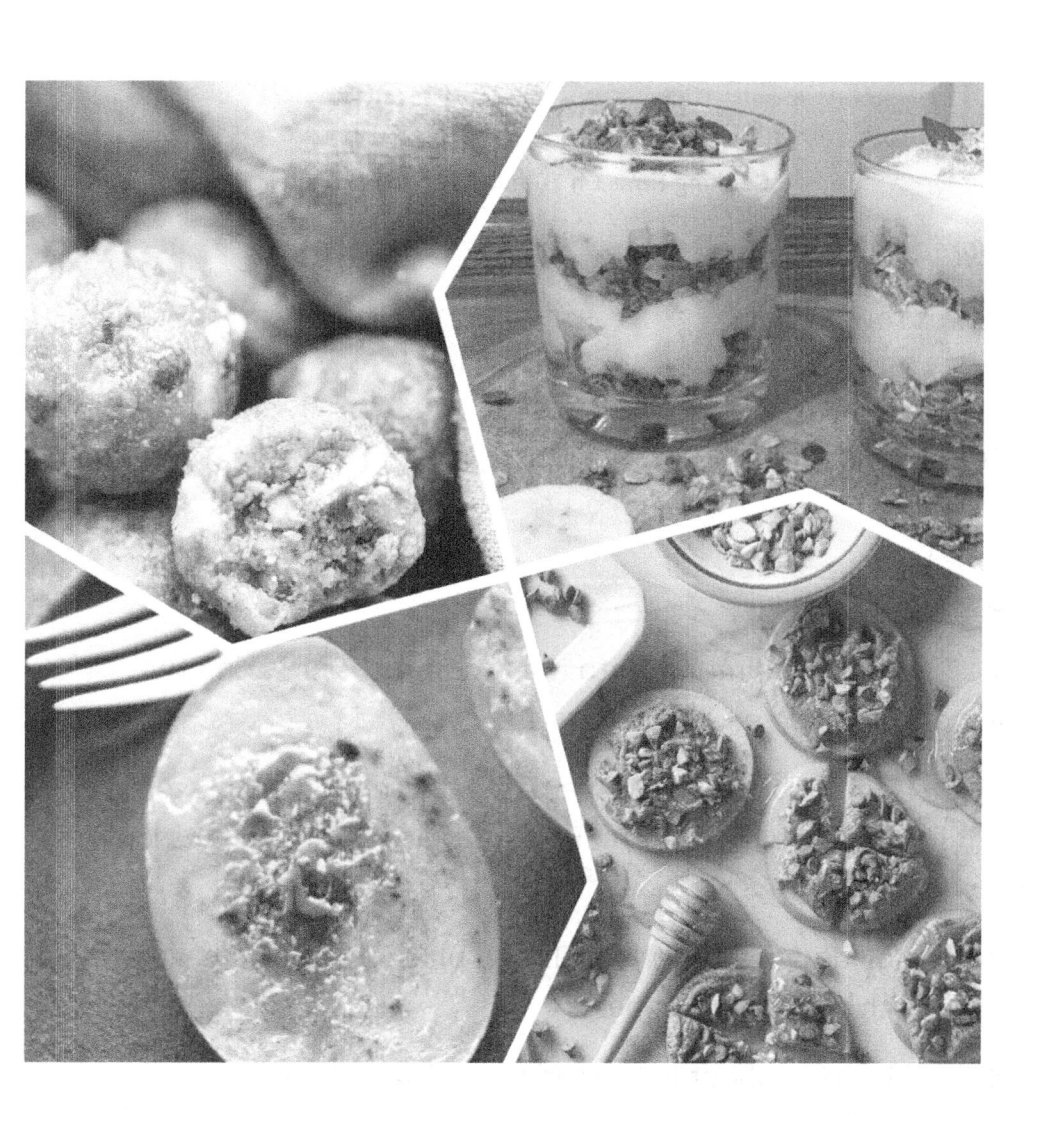

Banana Bread Bites

Cooking time 1 h 10 min| Servings 20 bites

Ingredients

2 cups raw almonds

1 ripe banana sliced

10-12 pitted dates

Directions

1.   Place the almonds into the food processor, grind the almonds into an excellent consistency.

2.   Add the banana and the dates to the food processor. Blend until a dough starts to form. Be sure that everything gets well combined.

3.   Roll dough into little balls and place them on a baking sheet lined with parchment paper.

4.   Place the sheet in the fridge for 1 hour.

Nutritional Facts per Serving (per bite): 298 calories, 7.8g protein, 23.1g fat, 16.3g carbohydrates.

Clean Eating Banoffee Parfaits

Cooking time 20 min| Servings 1

Ingredients

1 large ripe banana

1 1/2 cups plain yogurt

2/3 cup granola

Optional berries or bananas

Date caramel

1/3 cup dates

1/3 cup milk

Directions

1. Peel and cut the bananas into 1/4" thick coins.

2. Take three small glasses or jars—Lay 2 teaspoons of granola in each of them.

3. Then, place the banana pieces on the granola. Next step – pour dates, caramel, and yogurt on it.

4. Repeat the portions.

5. Finish with the rest of the ingredients to your taste.

Dates Caramel

1. Pit and chop the dates. Place them into a food processor.

2. Add milk, optional add salt. Blend the ingredients until smooth.

3. Pour the mixture into a saucepan. Cook stirring over low heat for 10 minutes until reduced down to 1/3 of the cup.

Nutritional facts per serving: 371 calories, 11.73g protein, 15g fat, 48.6g carbohydrates.

Mango and Cinnamon

Cooking time 10 min | Servings 4

Ingredients

2 mangos

1/4 cup turbinado sugar

1/8 tsp ground ginger

1/4 tsp ground cinnamon

pinch of ground nutmeg

Directions

1. Turn on the grill. Take the baking sheet and line it with foil.

2. Cut through the mango, remove the pit.

3. Take a small bowl, place sugar, ginger, cinnamon, nutmeg into it. Combine them generously sprinkle the mixture on top of mango slices.

4. Place the mango on the baking sheet, and broil until the sugar has caramelized, for 3-5 minutes.

Nutritional facts per serving: 159 calories, 0.9g protein, 0.55g fat, 30.6g carbohydrates.

Mini Fruit Pizzas

Cooking time 10 min | Servings 8

Ingredients

8 tbsp mini chocolate chips

4 tsp chopped salted roasted pistachios

1 apple

8 tbsp almond butter

4 tsp honey

Directions

1. Wash the apple, cut it into 8 pieces, slices. Remove the seeds.

2. Spread each portion of the apple with the butter, one tablespoon for each piece.

3. Chop the pistachios. Top the apple slices with nuts and honey.

Nutrition facts per serving: 180 calories, 4.2 g protein, 12.8 g fat, 16.3 g carbohydrates.

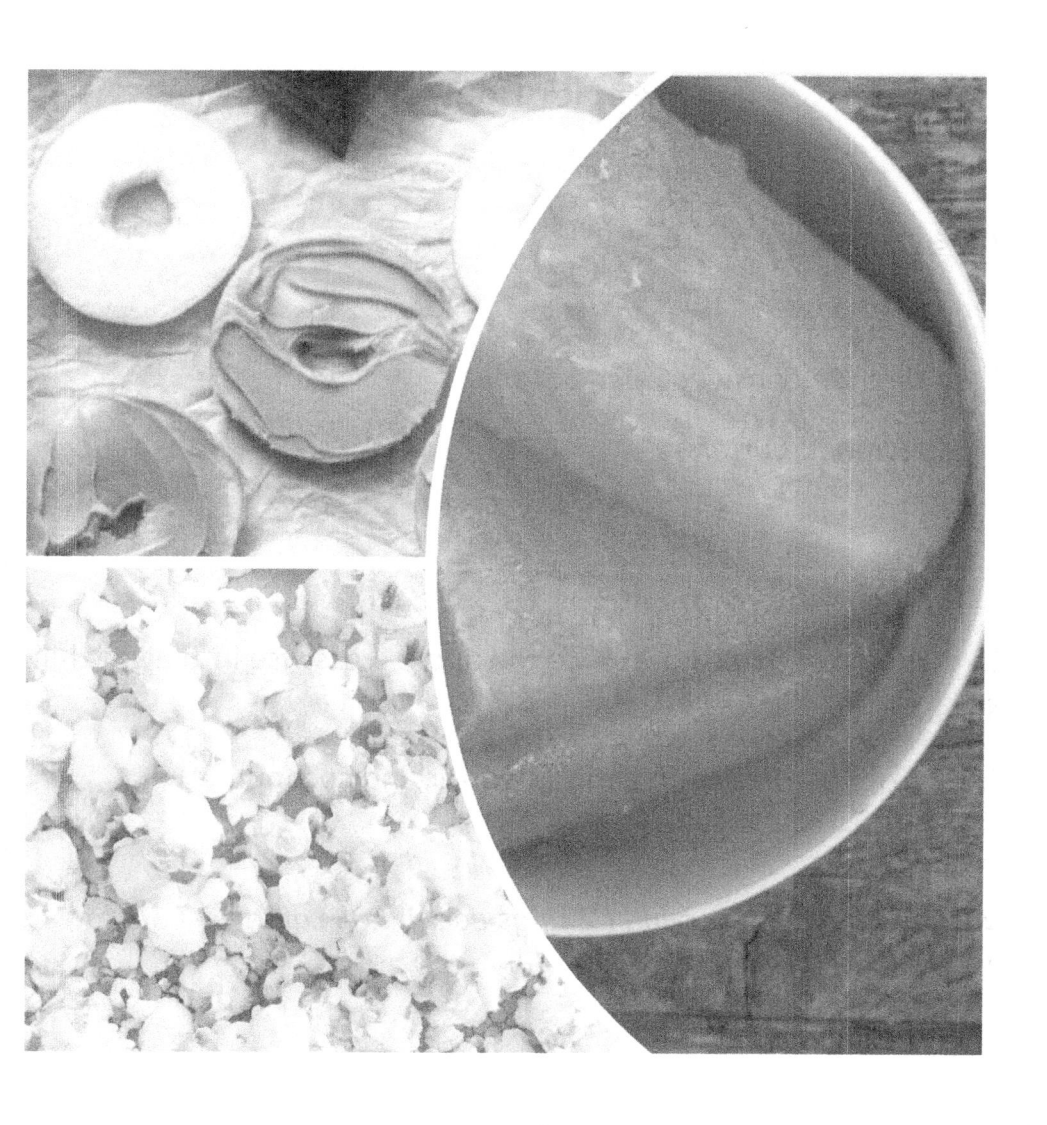

Apple "Donuts"

Cooking time 10 min | Servings 4

Ingredients

1 medium apple

2 tsp shredded unsweetened coconut

3 tbsp almond butter

Directions

1. Remove apple core. Slice the apple crosswise into eight thin rings.
2. Top the rings with almond butter and coconut.

Nutrition facts per serving (2 rings each): 103 calories, 7.3 g fat, 8.7 g carbohydrates, 2.7 g protein.

Birthday Cake Popcorn

Cooking time 15 min| Servings 8

Ingredients

2 tbsp popcorn kernels

2 tbsp white chocolate chips

½ tsp canola oil

1 tsp naturally dyed rainbow sparkling sugar

Directions

1. Take a brown paper bag, place popcorn kernels there, and fold the bag over three times.

2. Microwave the bag with kernels on 'High' for 3-4 minutes, microwave until popping stops.

3. Take a microwave-safe bowl, place chocolate chips in it. Microwave on "Medium" in 30-second until softened.

4. Add oil to the bowl with chocolate, stir the ingredients continuously until smooth.

5. Take a medium bowl, transfer the chocolate to it. Place the popcorn and sparkling sugar, toss until evenly coated.

Nutritional facts per serving (2 cups): 238 calories, 10.9 g fat, 35.1 g carbohydrates, 4.3 g protein.

Watermelon-Strawberry Popsicles

Cooking time 6 h 15 min | Servings 6

Ingredients

2 3/4 cups strawberries

2 cups cubed watermelon

¼ cup lime juice

2 tbsp light brown sugar

⅛ tsp salt

Directions

1. At first, slice ¾ cup strawberries. Take six 3-ounce freezer-pop molds. Press slices to the insides of them

3. Seed the watermelon, cube it.

4. In a food processor, place 2 cups of strawberries, pieces of watermelon, add lime juice, sugar, and salt. Blend the ingredients well.

5. Take the fine-mesh sieve, use it for cleaning the mixture. Pour the mixture through it into a medium bowl.

6. Pour the mixture into the molds, insert the sticks.

7. Place the molds into the freezer for about 6 hours.

Nutrition facts per serving: 57 calories; 0.3 g fat, 14.5 g carbohydrates, 0.8 g protein.

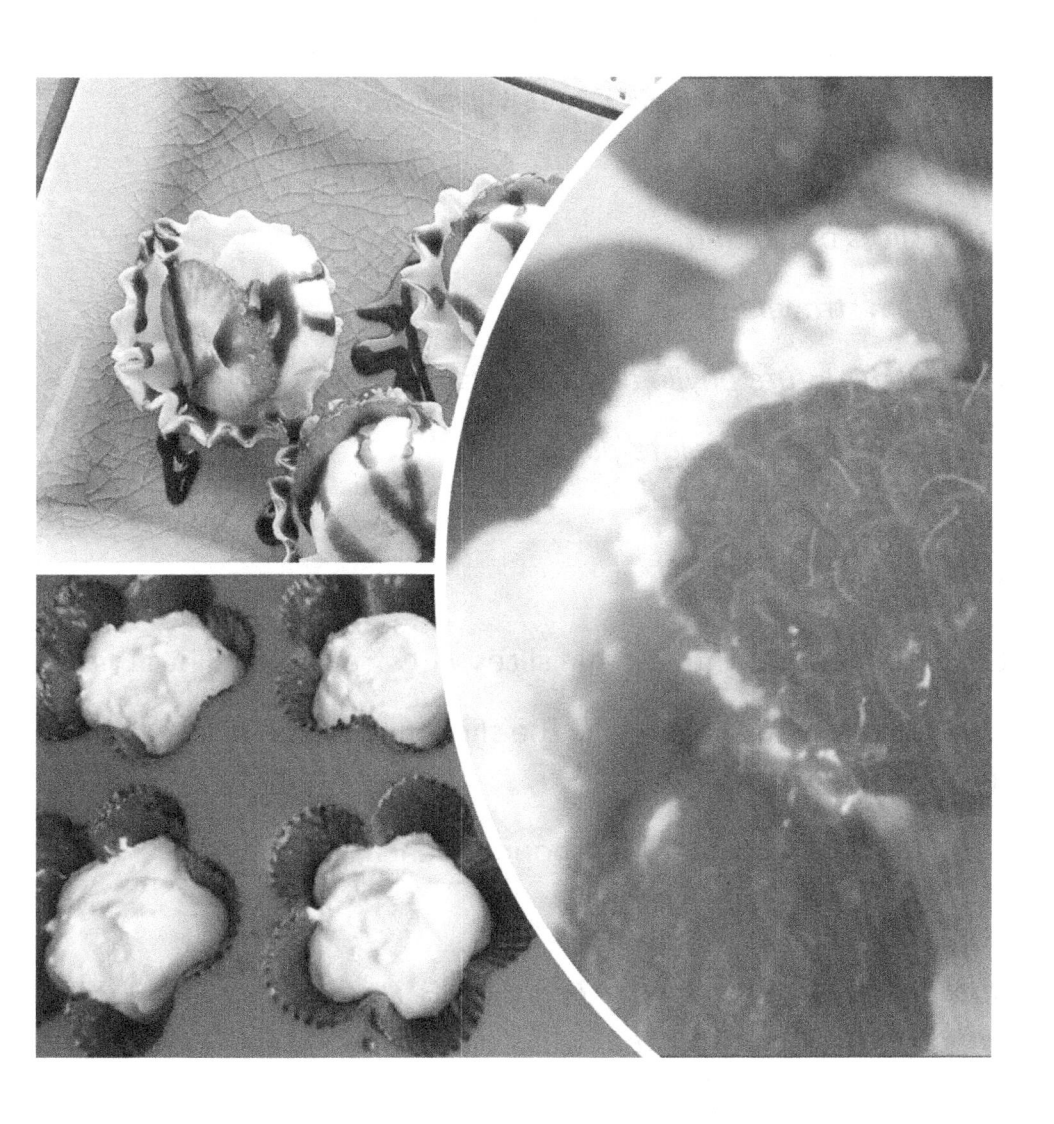

Banana Tarts

Cooking time 10 min | Servings 3

Ingredients

6 thin slices of banana

3 medium strawberry

6 baked miniature phyllo dough shells

3 tsp sugar-free chocolate-flavor syrup

Directions

1. Cut bananas into six thin slices, cut strawberries into thirds.

2. Take baked shells, place the slices and pieces of banana and strawberries in each shell.

3. Drizzle syrup, for ½ teaspoon for each shell.

Nutrition facts per serving: 67 calories, 3.1 g fat, 9.9 g carbohydrates, 0.2 g protein.

Ginger-Berry Dessert

Cooking time 10 min | Servings 1

Ingredients

¼ cup vanilla fat-free Greek yogurt

¼ cup fresh raspberries

1 gingersnap cookie

Directions

1. Take a small bowl, pour yogurt into it.
2. Crush the gingersnap cookies in a bowl. Add to the yogurt.
3. Top the dessert with raspberries.

Nutrition facts per serving: 88 calories, 0.9 g fat, 13.7 g carbohydrates, 6.5 g protein.

Lemon Cheesecake

Cooking time 2 hours| Servings 2

Ingredients

½ lb soft cream cheese

2 oz fatty cream

1 tbsp lemon juice

1 tsp stevia in liquid form

Vanilla to taste

Directions

1. Put cream cheese and cream in a bowl. Mix the ingredients with a mixer until uniform mass.

2. Add stevia, lemon juice, vanilla, lemon zest. Mix well.

3. Put the mixture into tart pans. You may consume it immediately. Chill in the refrigerator for two hours.

Nutritional facts per serving: 340 calories, 35 fat, 6g protein, 6g carbs

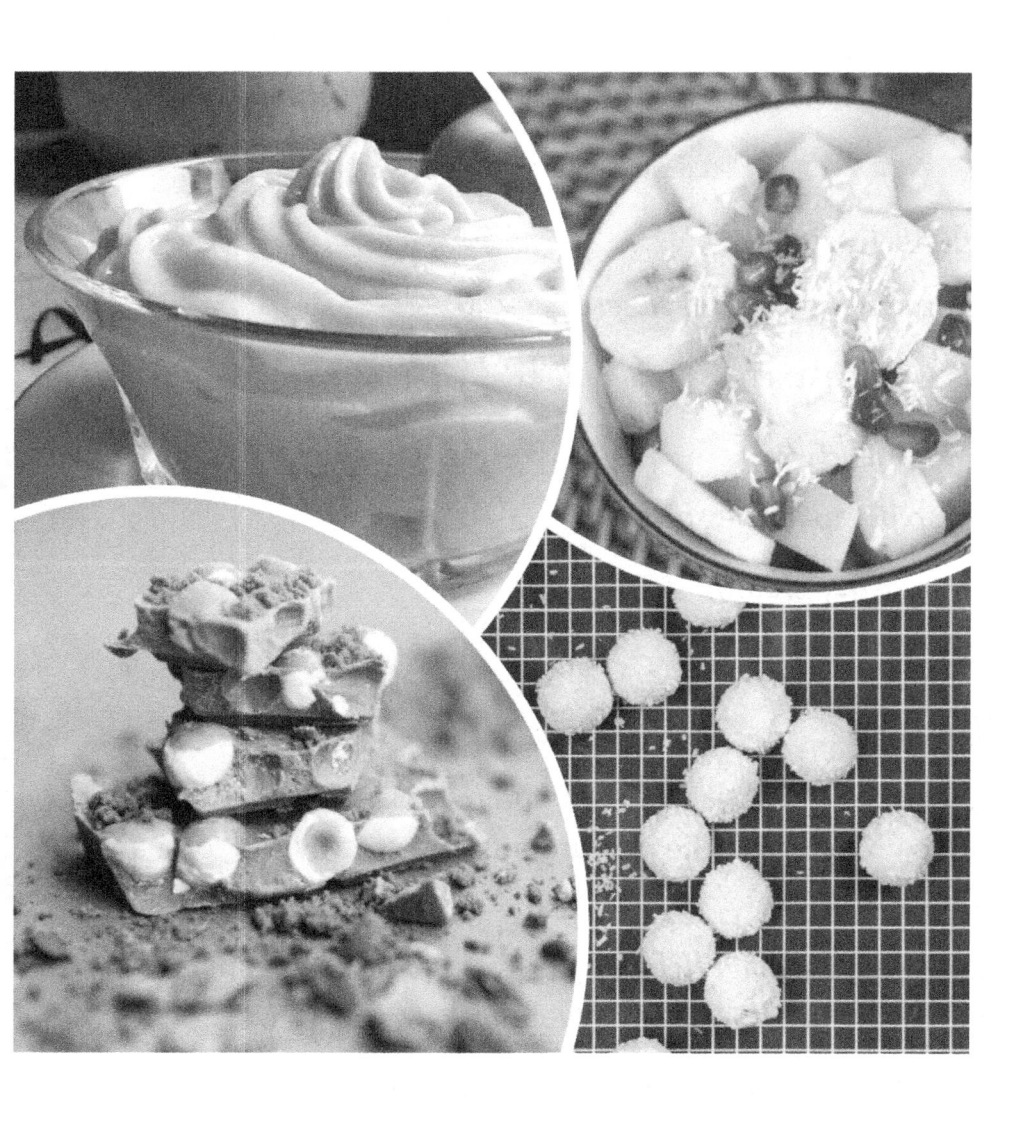

Pumpkin Cheesecake Mousse

Cooking time 2 hours| Servings 10

Ingredients

12 oz softened cream cheese

1 lb unsweetened pumpkin puree

½ cup erythritol

2 tbsp pumpkin pie spice

¾ cup heavy cream

Directions

1. Combine the cream cheese and pumpkin puree by hand in a large mixing bowl. The mixture must be creamy, smooth, and without clumps.

2.   Add vanilla, spices, erythritol, and heavy cream to the pumpkin mixture. Combine well.

3.   Refrigerate the mousse before serving.

Nutritional Facts per Serving: 173 calories, 15.3 g fat, 17.9 g carbs, 3.5 g protein

Tropical Fruits Salad

Cooking time 15 min | Servings 4

Ingredients

1 pineapple

2 mangoes

2 bananas

½ cup pomegranate seeds

2 tbsp sweet coconut shavings

Directions

1. Wash, peel, and cut pineapple, mango, and bananas into medium cubes. Put fruits on a deep plate.

2. Add the pomegranate seeds to the dish, mix, and let stand for several hours in the refrigerator.

3. Sprinkle with coconut flakes before eating.

Nutritional facts per serving: 350 calories, 2.5 g protein, 60 g carbs, 4.5 g fat.

Vegan Chocolate Turron

Cooking time 2 hours| Servings 16

Ingredients

9 oz dark chopped chocolate

2 tbsp melted coconut oil

1 ½ oz unsalted raw hazelnuts

Directions

1. Place dark chocolate in a saucepan. Cook over medium heat, occasionally stirring until chocolate is melted.

2. Remove chocolate from the heat. Add hazelnuts, and combine well.

3. Pour the chocolate-hazelnuts mixture into a lined rectangular dish.

4. Cool to room temperature. Chop the turron.

5. If it's too hot in the room, keep turron in the fridge.

Nutritional facts per serving: 128 calories, 1.3g protein, 9.9g carbs, 9.2g fat

Coconut Snowballs

Cooking time 15 min | Servings 2

Ingredients

3 oz shredded coconut

1 oz almond flour

2 ½ oz agave syrup

Directions

1. Mix 2 ounces of shredded coconut, flour, and syrup in a food processor until well combined.

2. Make ten balls using your hands.

3. Roll the balls in 1 ounce shredded coconut.

4. You can keep these balls in a sealed container in a fridge for one week.

Nutritional facts per serving: 398.5 calories, 6.2 g protein, 33.7 g carbs, 26.4 g fat

Made in the USA
Monee, IL
15 March 2025